INTRODUCTION

This concise but thorough handbook intended for the consumer, presents all of the most essential aspects of the American healthcare systems, services and products. It is updated and published annually, and mid-year, in order to incorporate any recent changes or perspectives. It is drawn from public sources and knowledge, both governmental and industry, to create an approachable and understandable overview. It is not presented as an in-depth academic work.

I hope this handbook shows you the path in your healthcare journey, through illness or enlightenment. Please reach out to me amadigiorgio@gmail.com if you find any inaccuracies or errors. I welcome any feedback.

Revised and Updated Version
March 26, 2021

Abbreviations

ACA	Affordable Care Act
ADA	Americans With Disabilities Act
ADN	Advanced Degree Nurse
CHIP	Children's Health Insurance Program
CMS	Center for Medicare and Medicaid Services
COBRA	Consolidated Omnibus Budget Reconciliation Act
CON	Certificate of Need
CPT	Current Procedural Terminology
EHR	Electronic Health Record
EI	Experimental and Investigational
EMR	Electronic Medical Record
EOB	Explanation of Benefits
ER	Emergency Room
ESRD	End Stage Renal Disease
FDA	U.S. Food and Drug Administration
FFS	Fee For Service
FRA	Full Retirement Age
FSA	Flexible Spending Account
HDHP	High Deductible Health Plan
HIPAA	Health Insurance Portability and Accountability Act
HHS	Health and Human Services
HSA	Health Savings Account
IRO	Independent Review Organization
ICD	International Classification of Diseases
LPN	Licensed Practical Nurse
LTC	Long-Term Care
OOP	Out Of Pocket
OTC	Over The Counter
P2P	Peer To Peer
PBM	Pharmacy Benefit Manager
PCA	Patient Care Assistant
PDP	Private Drug Plan
PPACA	Patient Protection and Affordable Care Act
QIO	Quality Improvement Organization
RBM	Radiology Benefit Manager
RN	Registered Nurse
SBC	Summary of Benefits and Coverage
SCHIP	State Children's Health Insurance Program
SNF	Skilled Nursing Facility
SSDI	Social Security Disability Insurance
SSI	Supplemental Security Income
TJC	The Joint Commission
UHC	United Health Care
VA	Veterans Affairs

U.S. HEALTHCARE PLANS

EMPLOYER-BASED HEALTHCARE

The United States healthcare system, with its delivery of medicine, is perceived domestically as the best in class. The U.S. spends twice as much on healthcare, compared to the other highest-income countries with similar population healthcare utilization. The U.S. also performs less favorable in population health outcomes. These include higher infant mortality, higher teen pregnancy and lower overall mortality. The U.S. ranks at the bottom twenty-five percentile for life expectancy. We have the highest motor vehicle deaths and gun homicides. We lead the world with more than 1/3 of our adult population as obese.

Some argue that our population, which is so much bigger than any one of these comparison countries, creates much greater challenges in population health. Adding to these disparities, the US has a higher comparative poverty rate. These are challenges. Ultimately, these challenges and statistics all translate to weak value for our national healthcare spending. The greatest and most fundamental contributor to this poor overall healthcare value being our high costs for healthcare goods and services. The major drivers to these increased costs are pharmaceuticals, medical devices and healthcare administrative services. These high costs occur even though the U.S. is the innovators in drug and medical device development and research. Since, we end up paying for these innovations. Each American individual spends about $1500 each year in pharmaceutical costs. This is twice per capita other developed countries.

There are many reasons Americans pay more for healthcare. One of the greatest healthcare service drivers of increased costs are high-margin, high-volume procedures, especially those involving joint or back surgeries. The procedure costs are compounded by adding the technical surgery costs to the high cost of the device or implant. Another reason for the increased US healthcare costs, is our aggressive litigious medico-legal environment. Many more malpractice cases are seen in the U.S. compared to other countries. The defensive medical practice, which is the provider doing more to avoid malpractice lawsuits, further drives up costs. Some have suggested well over half of all healthcare requests for tests and services, are attributed to non-value-added defensive medicine. Oftentimes, excess or over-utilization is blamed as a major driver to increased healthcare costs: doing services that do not need to be done. Admittedly, many of these are patient request based on advertising. Yet, efforts to change our utilization, by decreasing tests and procedures volume, seem to have had no real impact on lowering costs. In fact, adding fiscal intermediary gatekeeper processes, has been shown to mostly increase costs, by adding administrative costs to the provider. Our healthcare professionals, both clinical and administrative, as well as healthcare executives, earn salaries also greater than their international peers. A solution to get to the level of the other comparable countries 'healthcare budgets would be to somehow eliminate administrative costs and lower prices. Getting there politically and culturally, has been our greatest challenge.

In 1930, Americans spent $23 per person in healthcare. This was 3.5% of the Gross National Product (GDP). Eighty-five years later, in 2015, healthcare costs were $9536 per person and 15% of GDP. The U.S. spend on healthcare GDP was 17.8% in 2019 and is expected to climb by 5.5% each year to nearly 20% by 2027. It is anticipated that the future drivers of healthcare spending will be mostly due to new drug introductions. Healthcare costs are rising as more Baby Boomers age into requiring more services. Corporate profits are made untethered from improvements in health.

The history of modern healthcare insurance begins with the history of hospitals. Hospitals were once places where care was delivered only to the poor and indigent. During this early time, hospitals actually led to the spread of diseases. Thereafter, hospitals began a transformation with the advent of germ theory and the development of vaccines and antibiotics. Hospitals became places for quality and cutting-edge care. This was good for the care of the public, but not good for running a business. Hospitals were facing financial challenges, running on a model of pure fixed costs. An occupied bed paid the same no matter the treatment. An unoccupied bed received no revenue. Hospitals then solved that problem by offering insurance coverage. This was quickly followed by newly created health insurance companies that could not behave like traditional insurance. These health insurers, due to the strength and pressure from both the hospitals and the American Medical Association, had to emulate the then developed non-profit Blue Cross Blue Shield. In this way, hospitals were paid by insurers at cost-plus, in order to cover the fixed and variable costs of care and the costs of invested capital. Unfortunately, there was no incentive for hospitals to control costs, and hospitals costs per-patient per-day accelerated. These insurers paid for doctor services as "reasonable and customary." This led to further increased healthcare spending with doctors adding a few percentages to fees, in order to capture the highest payer. Yet, equilibrium was not reached through this structure of paying all hospital costs up to a certain level. It failed to adapt over time to the increasingly serious longer-term illnesses and expensive treatments that were becoming a dominant part of the growing hospital censuses. Major medical insurance stepped in, beginning around 1950, to supplement against catastrophic medical events and their explosive costs.

Employer-based health insurance arose during World War II. The labor market became tight, with 12 million American men serving in the armed forces. During this time, price controls restricted upward movement of wages, allowing only incentive recruitment. The Internal Revenue Service, IRS gave relief to companies by ruling health insurance tax-deductible for businesses. These companies were then able to use this employee health insurance as an additional hiring incentive. The National Labor Relations Board then decided in favor of health benefits under collective bargaining. Subsequently, labor unions demanded and won healthcare coverage during their negotiations. But, the burgeoning healthcare insurance market was bumpy. Health insurers were able to pick and choose to cover select and larger companies with reduced risk pooling. They left smaller business employees uncovered, as higher risk less profitable pools.

Medicare as healthcare for the elderly and Medicaid as healthcare for poor, was initially opposed by both hospitals and doctors. These federal healthcare programs were implemented in 1965, after agreeing to also model them like Blue Cross. This implementation led to an enormous surge in U.S. patients entering hospitals and being seen by providers. It was a major financial windfall for these stakeholders. The incomes of medical professionals doubled over the next decade. Not only did the Government became the largest insurer of healthcare in the U.S. but had tremendous political influence over the hospitals and providers. The financial windfalls came at the costs of governmental influence and intervention. This increase in both the medical care delivery and income of these providers led to a correlative increase in medical malpractice lawsuits. Increasing lawsuits led to mitigative changes in physician's practice styles: no-stone-unturned practice of defensive medicine.

There have been several important and beneficial changes to our modern healthcare system. The Affordable Care Act (ACA), also called "ObamaCare", was passed to increase healthcare access for uninsured and unemployed or employed without healthcare benefits. The ACA cut nearly in half those uninsured especially in states that expanded Medicaid. This individual ACA health plan, which is often subsidized, can be reviewed and subscribed via the web by anyone residing in any of the 50 states, through the state's HealthCare Exchange (healthcare.gov). The greatest benefit of the ACA legislation was removal of both pre-existing condition exclusions and maximum lifetime spends.

We are the only 1st world country without a national health plan. Reforms have been on and off political agendas for at least a century. First beginning with President Theodore Roosevelt before 1912 and more recently, "Medicare for All" during the last Democratic primaries. Reforms could also address the practice of doing more for more fees through the current and traditional Fee-for-Service (FFS) structure, by moving toward fixed payments for an episode of illness. Another potential reform that meets resistance from hospitals and insurers, is to create hospital price transparencies. Much of healthcare spending is on hospitals and professional services. Healthcare spending varies widely for the same service within the same city and across regions. Price transparency theoretically, allows patients to shop for lower-cost services, just as they do for an electric dryer or pair of shoes. Price transparency can also thwart surprise billing, which occurs when your insurer does not cover a portion or all of your care. This can happen when, for instance, a person is rushed to the nearest emergency room and the hospital or doctor is not "in-network." The patient is then personally responsible for that portion of that medical bill.

There has been strong opposition to U.S. healthcare care forms by the over 900 private health insurance companies which cover 2/3s of Americans. The average annual premium costs for the current year are nearly $8000 for an individual and over $20,000 for most families. Cost sharing has also been increasing and family Health Savings Account, HSA contributions can be as over $8000 per year. At the same time private health insurers have become increasingly profitable, sometimes garnering executive salaries over $20,000,000.

References and Links

https://www.healthaffairs.org/doi/10.1377/hlthaff.25.6.1538

https://journalofethics.ama-assn.org/article/us-health-care-non-system-1908-2008/2008-05

https://pnhp.org/a-brief-history-universal-health-care-efforts-in-the-us/

https://www.hhs.gov/healthcare/about-the-aca/index.html

COBRA

The Consolidated Omnibus Budget Reconciliation Act of 1986, referred to as COBRA, requires employers with at least 20 employees to provide a temporary extension of their employee health plan benefits to former employees as a non-subsidized full-priced plan. In other words, COBRA will cost what the employer and employee paid for that total health plan premium. It may be a lower-cost overall premium because of the negotiated rates, especially by larger employers. COBRA costs to the former employee may occasionally be subsidized by the employer. Certain former employees may be eligible for a refundable monthly premium payments through the Federal Health Coverage Tax Credit (HCTC). The HCTC pays 72.5% of qualified health insurance premiums for those who have lost their jobs due to the negative effects of global trade, the Trade Adjustment Assistance (TAA) Program or the Pension Benefit Guaranty Corporation (PBGC).

COBRA health coverage can begin on the date after termination and last up to 18 months. The termination can be by resignation, being fired, retirement, losing work hours or because a dependent aging out of their employment group health plan. COBRA can extend to 36 months for the spouse or ex-spouse due to the death of a former employee, divorce from the former employee, or the aging into Medicare of the former employee. Most states allow COBRA for even longer periods of time, beyond 18 months. This state continuation coverage, also called "mini-COBRA." This extension may be for a few to several more months, under certain conditions, such as disability and/or require higher premium (for example 115%) payments.

The employer is required to notify the health plan administrator within 30 days of any employee termination. The employee must receive notice from the plan administrator within another 14 days. The employer has the full 44 days if they are also the health plan administrator. Each qualified beneficiary on that former employee health plan receives notification of their right to elect COBRA coverage. This notice will include such important information as the monthly premium amount and the date the election for COBRA acceptance needs to be made. The election needs to be made by 60 days from the time of notice. COBRA coverage, if chosen, will be retroactive to the date after termination. There is a 2% administration fee added to the monthly premium costs of COBRA. If COBRA is not elected, this will trigger a 60 days special enrollment period within the ACA exchange. Some states extended this special enrollment period even further during the COVID outbreak. The present Administration plans to open ACA enrollment up again in mid-2021. COBRA is expensive, because group health insurance and private health insurance is expensive. COBRA is often a good bridge to an ACA plan or when becoming Medicare eligible. Some former employees or dependents may also meet eligibility and immediately transition to Medicaid or Medicare. COBRA also gives the former employee and dependents a bridge until the next employment or other sources of healthcare. Many former employees continue with COBRA on termination, because they have already met a level of cost sharing for that plan year, toward meeting the total out-of-pocket annual spend. Otherwise, a new plan cost-sharing would otherwise start from scratch. COBRA has been an effective way for former employees to maintain healthcare while transitioning to the next source of coverage.

References and Links
https://www.dol.gov/general/topic/health-plans/cobra
https://www.healthcare.gov/unemployed/cobra-coverage/

AFFORDABLE CARE ACT

There is a large proportion of Americans working lower wage jobs, whose employers do not offer benefits, including healthcare. Or the employers offer only simple benefits that do not include healthcare insurance. These are primarily small businesses, food industries and "gig" workers (Airbnb, TaskRabbit, Uber, etc.). The uninsured rate in the US has hovered around 15% for decades. Healthcare received by these uninsured individuals is primarily during crisis or accident and delivered through the Emergency Room (ER). Preventive care is mostly absent. There are a number of studies which show that the uninsured don't live as long as those who are insured. They have higher rates of progressive chronic illnesses and higher mortality from cancer.

The Patient Protection and Affordable Care Act (PPACA) was passed in 2010. This allowed anyone not covered by their employer or not covered by a government health program (Medicare, Medicaid, CHIP, etc.) to buy a Gold, Silver or Bronze individual health plan, through their state exchange. The state exchanges are accessed on www.healthcare.gov. These health plans are subsidized according to income, cover pre-existing conditions and have no annual maximum benefit amount.

This legislation has nearly cut in half those uninsured. Open enrollment into one of these individual or family plans varies by state, but is typically November 1st to December 15th. The coverage then starts effective January 1st of the following year. Special enrollment can occur through the year if there is the loss of a job, a marriage or the birth of a baby. Special enrollment can also occur if you will lose COBRA or if your employer stopped contributing premium to your COBRA. FEMA had extended Special Coverage enrollment beyond 60 days due to the national emergency of COVID-19. The current Administration will do this again this year. Special enrollment can also occur if an "exceptional circumstance," serious medical condition, natural disaster, or other national or state-level emergency, kept one from enrolling.

It should be noted that ACA was not the first attempt to develop a public option or universal coverage. President Theodore Roosevelt discussed universal coverage during his term in office. He was, however, not re-elected in 1912 in order to carry this out. But his distant cousin did make a huge step forward for the American people. President Franklin D. Roosevelt signed the Social Security Act in 1935. Roosevelt's healthcare plan enactment was passed to the vice president, then President Harry Truman, upon Roosevelt's death. Truman's universal healthcare Wagner-Murray-Dingell Bill never made it to a vote. Lyndon Johnson won a landslide 1964 election and quickly enacted Medicare and Medicaid, before his political capital waned. In contrast, the Clinton administration waited until his second term in 1993, before beginning deliberations on healthcare reform. This failed attempt was blamed for the turnover from that Democratic controlled Congress. Presidents Nixon, Eisenhower, Kennedy, Carter and George W Bush (Medicare Pharmacy) all considered, attempted, and some had success, in healthcare reforms. There is significant tension currently in any attempts to broader American healthcare coverage through a single or governmental plan, between their advocates and the strong deep-pockets healthcare lobby. The ACA was intended as an initial, albeit broadly impacting, step toward a public accessible healthcare option for the people of America. It has survived through rancor and passion.

References and Links
https://www.hhs.gov/healthcare/about-the-aca/index.html
https://www.kff.org/wp-content/uploads/2011/03/5-02-13-history-of-health-reform.pdf

HEALTH SHARE

Health Sharing plans, also called Medical Sharing Societies, Medical Cost-Sharing Organizations, Medical Sharing Networks and Bill Sharing are an alternative to formal health insurance. Members submit monthly premiums, or "shares" which are then pooled and redistributed or "shared" to other members for eligible medical expenses. The sharing is done through administration of the plan. A few plans have the sharing for medical expenses, directly member to member. Their premiums are lower than conventional group or individual insurances, because coverage is more restricted. They are not supervised under the ACA and therefore are not required to cover pre-existing conditions, do not have a lifetime maximum and not truly open to all participants of religion and background. Health sharing has been around since 1993, beginning with the Melbourne Florida based, Midi-Share. Health sharing have gained in popularity, more recently, for those groups that are more Christian religious, more conservative, and opposed to the ACA structure. Health shares do not use actuaries, do not accept risk or make guarantees of payment and do not purchase re-insurance. But they do allow lower cost negotiation with providers and facilities, through cash payments. Their version of deductibles are called "unshare amounts", "share amounts" or "family share amounts." Many states have enacted safe harbor laws for health share plans, so they do not need to be regulated as insurance. As a consequence, the premiums are not tax deductible. About 1 million Americans belong to a health sharing ministry. Health shares currently administer about ¾ of a billion dollars in medical bills.

Health sharing, in the majority of these products, requires a connection to Christianity and its congregations. In fact, federal inclusion as a 501(c)(3) organization and exemption from the ACA requires members to "share common ethical or religious beliefs." Some health shares require the community pastor or leader to verify the member's beliefs, or confirm attendance quotas. The health share Aliera is open to all religious groups. There is a Jewish health sharing organization, United Refuah. Another health share, Sedera Health, only requires the member to "live a healthy lifestyle." Most health shares require acknowledgment against, and will terminate the coverage with, excessive alcohol consumption, smoking or the abuse of drugs and even extra-marital sex. Many do not cover birth control, abortions or risky behavior, such as rock climbing or motorcycle driving without a helmet. There is no coverage for self-inflicted injury or any ambulance benefit. Most do cover tele-health, which is becoming more mainstream, even with conventional health plans. Very few cover pre-existing conditions. Expensive prescriptions are covered up to a limit. Maintenance medications are usually fully covered. Many health shares allow choosing your own provider. There are no free wellness visits nor preventative care, as required under the ACA. Some will support additional premiums for catastrophic coverage. Most have a lifetime maximum. There is generally no open enrollment time. In other words, application for coverage can be sought throughout the year.

Probably the biggest drawback to Health Shares, is getting payment reimbursement for rendered healthcare services. Some health shares will negotiate directly with the provider. But many leave that to you. In other words, the patient is on the hook for the full fee and get reimbursed by the Health Share for a certain amount. Hospitals are not either familiar with or embrace these unregulated products. They are often wary of accepting them as guarantee of payment for hospital admission. So, the member will have to leave a deposit or personal guarantee of payment before receiving hospital treatments. Hospitals may not be accepting of the discounted payment offered by the Health Shares. Anyone considering these programs should fully scrutinize them, since the lower costs are also associated with they an unregulated product, focused on certain members, deliver limited benefits and have a unique process for payments.

References and Links
https://www.calhealth.net/pros-and-cons-of-health-sharing-plans-like-alieracare.htm
https://www.clarkscondensed.com/alternative-health-insurance-options-health-share-comparison/

SHORT-TERM HEALTH INSURANCE

Short-term health plans have many features comparable with Health Sharing, including no open enrollment period, lower premiums and choice of providers. They are also similar with the lack of broad coverage or coverage for pre-existing conditions. Similarly, they don't cover routine office visits and many don't cover every-day prescriptions. Short-term health insurance are basic underwriting plans. Although described as "short" term plans, many are getting even longer, competing with ACA-compliant health plans. Yet, they are not available in all states. Short-term health insurance is oriented toward those healthy individuals or families living in states without Medicaid expansion, or those that find conventional ACA health plans unaffordable.

The Obama Administration, during the ACA roll-out, shortened these short-term plans from a duration of under one year, to less than three months. They were positioned as a stop-gap until another ACA or group plan was restarted. They were concerned that those low-risk jumping into short-term plans could destabilize the ACA market. The Trump Administration, on October 2, 2018, reversed this to allow up to 364 days on these short-term plans, and even added on renewals up to 36 months. The Biden Administration has discussed rolling back some of these short-term plan expansions. A short-term health plan should be considered just that: restricted health coverage for a limited period as a bridge to a full-coverage plan.

References and Links
https://www.healthaffairs.org/do/10.1377/hblog20190720.616648/full/ (Court Upholds Short Term Health Insurance)

MEDICARE

Medicare can be broad and complicated. The individual needs to be aware of the benefits and pitfalls of its policies, including enrollment timelines and requirements. President Lyndon B. Johnson signed the Social Security Amendments of 1965, creating both Medicare and Medicaid. Medicare is a national health insurance program, initially oriented toward those 65 or older. Medicare includes those under 65 and disabled, and any age with End-Stage Renal Disease (ESRD) requiring dialysis or a kidney transplant. In addition, the Medicare program includes benefits for spouses and dependents. Medicare core coverage and benefits are divided into parts A, B, C and D, depending on the category of healthcare. These parts often include member cost-sharing requirements. You need to sign up to get Medicare Part A (Hospital Insurance) and Part B (Medical Insurance) beginning 3 months before turning 65. The complete 7-month window to sign up, in addition to the 3 months before, also includes the one month you turn 65, and the following 3 months. For example, a prospective Medicare beneficiary can sign up on January 1st if their birthday is on April 1st and no later than July 31st. On August 1st, you are considered late. You won't get Medicare automatically. Automatic Medicare Part A and Part B occurs if the beneficiary is already getting benefits from Social Security, such as Social Security Disability or ESRD.

Do not delay signing up for Medicare. You will likely incur penalties if you do not enroll in Medicare when first eligible. The Medicare Part A penalty is an additional 10% of your monthly premium, regardless of the length of the delay. You have to pay this higher premium for twice the number of years of the delay (i.e., two years of premium penalty for a one-year delay). The Medicare Part B late-enrollment penalty could span for as long as you have Medicare Part B. The penalty goes up 10% for every 12-month period you didn't enroll in Part B (i.e., 3-year delay increases premium by 30%). The late-enrollment penalty for Medicare Prescription Drug Plans is calculated by multiplying 1% of the "national base beneficiary premium" by the number of months you were eligible and added to your monthly prescription drug plan premium. This penalty may stretch the whole time enrolled in a Medicare Prescription Drug Plan.

Medicare Part A is referred to as the Medicare Hospital Insurance, which mainly includes inpatient hospital care, but also includes critical access hospitals, short-term skilled-nursing facility care, hospice and home healthcare. Most beneficiaries don't pay a Part A premium for Part A since they, or their spouse, has already paid for it through their employment payroll taxes. This is called "Premium-free Part A." These premium-free groups include those at 65 or their spouses who have paid Medicare taxes for at least 10 years, those under 65 and disabled receiving Social Security benefits or Railroad Retirement Board disability benefits for two years, have ESRD receiving dialysis, and either you or your spouse or parent (if you're a dependent child) who has paid Medicare taxes for at least 10 years or have amyotrophic lateral sclerosis (ALS) while eligible for

Social Security Disability Insurance (SSDI) as long as you or your spouse (or parent, if you're a dependent child) paid Medicare taxes for at least 10 years. All others will have to pay a premium of about $250-450 per month.

Medicare Part B, also called Medical Insurance, covers what is considered outpatient care. These include doctors' office services, physical and occupational therapy, some other types of home healthcare, laboratory tests and medical supplies. Most members pay a monthly premium for Part B. This premium is currently under $200 for those with no income or lower income. Higher levels of income require higher premiums.

Parts A and B delivered directly through the federal government's Center for Medicare and Medicaid Services (CMS), are referred to as "original" or "traditional" Medicare. Most people use this Medicare traditional fee-for-service program. The traditional Medicare member can use any doctor and hospital that takes Medicare. The member does pay co-insurance for some services and the provider must accept what Medicare pays for that service. This does not require subscription through a health plan. Parts A and B can also be delivered through a Medicare Advantage plan or can be supplemented with Medigap insurance. Funds are allocated to these private insurance plans, who then administer the Medicare coverages.

Medicare Part C is always delivered by Medicare Advantage plans. Medicare Advantage are private health plans that must provide all Part A and Part B services covered by traditional Medicare. But they can do so with different rules, costs, and restrictions. One restriction may be their requirement for use of in-network providers and facilities. These Medicare Advantage administered plans would, therefore, not include all providers and facilities under traditional Medicare. Another restriction could be the requirement for referral or authorization in order to receive care. This step would not be required under traditional Medicare. Like private health plans under the ACA, Medicare Advantage plans may have annual limits on out-of-pocket costs. You will have to pay a premium to receive coverage and also have cost-sharing. Medicare Advantage plans can provide additional benefits that traditional Medicare does not cover, such as routine vision or dental care. Dental and vision care are rarely part of a private health plan, and you will likely pay a hired premium for these additional benefits.

Medicare Part D is the Prescription Drug Coverage portion of Medicare. Part D prescription drug coverage requires subscribing to a plan approved by Medicare that offers Medicare drug coverage. This can either be through the Medicare Advantage plan or, if keeping traditional Medicare, joining a stand-alone Medicare private drug plan (PDP). Medicare drug plans differ in costs and formularies. Most people pay a monthly premium for Part D. A premium penalty, later on, may be imposed if you do not sign up for a Part D plan when eligible.

The Medicare Part D "donut hole", or Coverage Gap, can occur if you meet a total-drug-costs amount for the year to date, as a member of a Part D PDP. Reaching this threshold amount leads to a higher cost member paying interval. This higher cost period was originally called a donut hole, because the member had to pay all the prescription costs. Now the member reaching this threshold instead pays a higher prescription co-pay amount. The fabled donut hole is now considered "closed." This higher prescription cost-sharing period begins at the Initial Coverage Limit. Then the higher cost sharing continues until the next January 1, or until out-of-pocket costs qualify you for Catastrophic Coverage. The Initial Coverage Limit in 2020 is $4,020 in total costs for the member's medications. From this point the member pays the higher cost-sharing described, until the total out-of-pocket costs reach the maximum of $6,350. The Catastrophic Coverage then begins. This out-of-pocket maximum includes the cost sharing but does not include health plan premiums, the cost of non-covered drugs, nor out-of-network pharmacy drug costs. These excluded costs are similar to private health plans. Only a small amount of the cost for drugs will be paid during Catastrophic Coverage.

Private supplemental insurance, called Medigap, can pay deductibles, co-insurances, and co-payments. Medigap has a long history, predating Medicare Advantage plans, and is still widely purchased today. There are 10 different Medigap plans to choose from (most called A, B, C, D, F, G, K, L, M, and N) offering both differing premiums and benefit sets. Medigap tends to give more flexibility than

Advantage plans in choice of provider and coverage while traveling. They also allow those who want to keep traditional Medicare some relief from its cost sharing. There are other ways to fill gaps in Medicare coverage or costs. Employment-based health insurance from you or your spouse may be primary or secondary to Medicare. Primary insurance pays first. A secondary insurance pays after the primary, if at all. Retiree insurance, sometimes offered to retired employees, always pays secondary. Veterans Affairs (VA) healthcare benefits and services may exceed those offered by Medicare, and can be less costly. Medicare does not pay for any VA care.

Those on Medicare with limited income may be eligible for Medicaid to pay Medicare co-pays and deductibles and care not offered by Medicare. Federal government run Medicare Savings Programs (MSPs) help pay the monthly Medicare Part B premium for those with limited ability to pay full premiums. Another program, the Qualified Medicare Beneficiary (QMB) program covers deductibles and coinsurances. The federal program, Part D Low-Income Subsidy (LIS) and referred to as "Extra Help," will pay for some or most of the costs of Medicare Part D prescription drug coverage. Enrollment in an MSP can automatically lead to enrollment in Extra Help. There are also some State Pharmaceutical Assistance Programs (SPAP) that assist with prescription costs.

References and Links
https://www.medicare.gov/
https://www.ssa.gov/benefits/medicare/

MEDICAID

Prior to the introduction of Medicaid and Medicare in 1965, federal money was granted to and used by the states to support their various public assistance programs. These programs were colloquially called "welfare." Medicaid was created under Title XIX of the Social Security Act, at the same time as the Medicare program (Title XVIII). Medicaid became a federal program that would distribute funds to pay at least half of core medical services to the states' indigent. Over 65 million people in the US are on Medicaid today. The states have the option to expand from these core healthcare services, even to those not receiving public assistance. Medicaid has developed coverage, over the years since inception, beyond healthcare services for the indigent, to now become the main support for long-term services for people with disabilities and nursing-home care. In 1972, Medicaid for people with disabilities was linked to Social Security Income (SSI) eligibility, only to be uncoupled from SSI eligibility in the late 1990s. The next decade brought more Medicaid coverage for mothers giving birth, de-institutionalized people with disabilities and began the use of managed care to control Medicaid healthcare costs.

The State Children's Health Insurance Program (SCHIP) was created in 1997 to extend Medicaid services to children in low-income households. That year also saw, through the Balanced Budget Act of 1997, new options for states to implement managed care approaches without having to seek special waivers. The Affordable Care Act of 2014 allowed states to expand Medicaid eligibility to individuals under age 65 in families with incomes below 133-138% of the Federal Poverty Level (FPL) and standardized the eligibility and benefits through Medicaid, CHIP and the Health Insurance Marketplace.

References and Links

https://www.medicaid.gov/

DUAL-ELIGIBLE

There are over 12 million beneficiaries who are "dual-eligible" for both Medicare and Medicaid benefits. In order to be dual-eligible one needs to qualify for both: Medicare because of age or disability and Medicaid based on the state's eligibility rules. The dual-eligible individual receives traditional Medicare Parts A and B and full state Medicaid benefits. The member is "full dual-eligible" by receiving full Medicaid and full Medicare benefits and is therefore not considered "partial dual-eligible." There are many categories of those less than full dual eligible, including those that are in the Qualified Medicare Beneficiary (QMB) Program, Specified Low-Income Medicare Beneficiary (SLMB) Program, Qualifying Individual (QI) Program and Qualified Disabled Working Individual (QDWI) Program, with varying eligibilities and benefits. The majority of duals are disabled and receive full benefits. Dual-eligibles can get their benefits through a Dual Special Needs plan (D-SNP). These plans include all the Medicaid and traditional Medicare Part A and Part B benefits, as well as Part D prescription drug coverage. These plans often include additional benefits, such as dental, vision and hearing coverage, health products purchase credits, and transportation assistance, at no extra cost.

References and Links
https://www.cms.gov/Medicare-Medicaid-Coordination/Medicare-and-Medicaid-Coordination/Medicare-Medicaid-Coordination-Office/Downloads/MMCO_Factsheet.pdf

CHILDREN'S HEALTH INSURANCE PLAN

The Children's Health Insurance Programs (CHIP), also called State Children's Health Insurance Program (SCHIP) was introduced in 1997 as an entitlement and block grant program to health insure children from families with too much income to qualify for Medicaid, but not enough to afford private insurance. This sweet-spot is about 100%–200% of the federal poverty level. The states can either provide this through Medicaid, a separate state administered program, or a combination of the two. Benefits must meet certain set standards and allow some flexibility in each state. State payments for child health assistance under SCHIP qualify for federal matching payments. This is just like Medicaid. The federal government pays 70% of SCHIP program costs, while the state pitches in the other 30%. Yet, these federal matching payments are limited by national and state-specific or annual limits on federal funding. The SCHIP program will redistribute some of the individual state unspent federal funds, to other states. By 2000, every state and the District of Columbia had children enrolled in SCHIP. This encompasses nearly 10 million children enrolled in SCHIP.

References and Links
https://www.benefits.gov/benefit/607

HEALTHCARE PRODUCTS

DISABILITY

There are two types of disability insurance and benefits. Which are administered through either private disability insurance carriers or the federal government's Social Security Disability Insurance (SSDI) program. More than 14 million Americans receive disability benefits through SSDI. There are far fewer receiving benefits through a private plan. Up to 15% of the American population, over 400 million people, is therefore on disability today. Over 90% of those disabled are former workers. Those receiving disability benefits are no longer counted in the U.S. workforce and therefore not added to the unemployment count. Applications for disability go up with unemployment and with the loss of state welfare benefits. Disabled residents of each state can vary widely. West Virginia is the highest (9%), while Utah, Hawaii and Alaska are the lowest (3%). Back pain and mental illness are the fastest growing causes of disability in adults. While, the number of children on disability has quadrupled in the last 20 years. Disability can come down to the doctor's opinion and clerical, administrative or judicial judgment.

About 1/3 of employees in the U.S. are offered private disability insurance. Many others purchase supplemental disability insurance on their own. Both groups use this private disability insurance to protect against loss of income. Private disability plans cover more definitions of disability than SSDI. These private plans protect against disability from either "own occupation" or "any occupation." These plans usually require the inability to do any work, in order to show total disability. The private plans will cover a greater share of the lost salary, when compared to SSDI benefits. One can qualify for both private and SSDI disability. However, the private disability pay-out may be deducted from the SSDI payment. Workers' Compensation and Veterans benefits can still be collected while receiving private disability and SSDI benefits. Yet, Workers' Compensation from a federal government job will reduce the SSDI payment.

There are two sections of the 1973 Rehabilitation Act which are important for disability rights. Section 501 supports people with disabilities in either federal workplaces or places receiving federal tax dollars. Section 504 prohibits discrimination against individuals with disabilities in any workplace and in their programs and activities. The regulations for Section 504 were not implemented until 1977. The Americans with Disabilities Act (ADA) of 1990 and the Amendments to this Act in 2008, were the major turning points against discrimination toward the disabled, in nearly all remaining aspects of life. Getting to this historic point was nevertheless tumultuous.

The passage of Social Security in 1935 completely left out disability insurance. At that time, there was difficulty on agreeing when an applicant was too disabled for work and concern over the potentially high cost to administer such a program. Yet, SSDI did become law in 1956. SSDI started off by allowing disability benefits to those disabled at age 50-64 or to their adult children with a disability beginning before the age of 18. Disability was defined as the "inability to engage in any substantial gainful activity by reason of any medically determinable physical or mental impairment which can be expected to result in death or to be of long-continued and indefinite duration." Today, SSDI covers those who have earned 40 Social Security work credits, half of these earned in the last 10 years. Each credit is about $1200 in salary. One cannot receive benefits until disabled for 5 months. Eligibility leads to an average monthly SSDI benefit of about $1200. SSDI is calculated at the beneficiary's full retirement amount. SSDI then transitions from disability to retirement status at the Full Retirement Age (FRA) of the beneficiary. So, in this way the benefit does not change during this disability to retirement transition. One can apply for SSDI after age 65 and before FRA, but with additional scrutiny by the federal government.

SSDI requires total disability and not partial or short-term disability. Social Security defines disability as the inability to do work that you did before, cannot adjust to other work and the disability has lasted or will last for at least one year or to result in death. There are some conditions that are deemed total disability without proof of disability. These include blindness, acute leukemia, Lou Gehrig's disease (ALS), and pancreatic cancer. All others must meet the disorder criteria published by Social Security in their "Listing Of Impairments," also called their "Blue Book."

Typical radiating back pain is the most common reason for SSDI. The "List of Impairments" in "Adult Listing Part A", under "1.00 Musculoskeletal System

44

1.04A." requires radiating pain with evidence of motor loss, either sensory or reflex loss and a positive straight-leg raising test to meet total disability. This is how an eligible disability, under SSDI, is evaluated and determined.

References and Links
https://www.ssa.gov/disability/

HEALTH SAVINGS ACCOUNT (HSA)

Health Savings Accounts (HSA) and Flexible Spending Accounts (FSA) were first introduced in 2004 as part of the Medicare Prescription Drug Improvement and Modernization Act. These arose because of the concern that "over-insurance" was leading to higher healthcare costs. In other words, overuse of healthcare benefits because they were unlinked from financial pain. This was believed that excessive medical spending could be reduced by the consumer directly controlling healthcare spending. Feeling the pain of healthcare costs.

The HSA arose as a better version of the predecessor Internal Revenue Service's piloted Archer Medical Savings Accounts (MSA). The HSA improved on the MSA concept by allowing members covered by High-Deductible Health Plans (HDHPs) to save on eligible expenses with the triple-tax advantages. The three tax advantages with HSAs are (1) contributions are pre-tax and tax-free, (2) account balances grow tax-free and (3) withdrawals on eligible expenses are also tax-free.

The ACA improved access to HDHPs, particularly for those without traditional coverage through their employers. The employer often contributes some portion of the members HSA annual amount. The total annual HSA contribution requirements increase going from an individual to a family plan and also increases with beneficiaries age 55 or older. HSA medical expenses can be reimbursed in any taxable year. Some approaching retirement use the funds in an HSA account to pay future eligible health expenses.

The IRS limits on contributions for each year, as well as eligible expenses can be found on the IRS website at the following link: https://www.irs.gov/publications/p969#en_US_2019_ publink1000204083. The CARES Act expanded eligible expenses for HSAs and FSAs to feminine hygiene products, over-the-counter (OTC) medications and tele-health appointments.

FLEXIBLE SPENDING ACCOUNT (FSA)

The Flexible Spending Account (FSA), which also has a tax-free contribution and distribution, is linked with an employment health plan. An FSA pays co-payments, deductibles, some drug costs, including eligible over-the-counter health items. The FSA pays some other healthcare costs, including dental. Using an FSA can reduce your taxes. A contribution portion toward the FSA can also come annually from the employer. The FSA contribution allowed increases from single status to married and family.

The FSA money must be used in that plan year, otherwise it is lost. Generally, you can't treat insurance premiums as qualified medical expenses for either the HSA or FSA. But, you can use HSA funds to pay premiums if collecting federal or state unemployment benefits, or COBRA coverage. The IRS publishes a list of eligible medical expenses, including those that apply to FSAs. This list can be found at https://www.irs.gov/publications/p502.

LONG-TERM CARE INSURANCE

Long-term care insurance can be helpful, since people are living longer. Increasing longevity increases the need for senior care. Long-term care insurance should cover any long-term need, such as home care, assisted living, adult daycare, respite care, hospice care, nursing homes, memory care facilities, and home modification to accommodate disabilities.

There are two types of long-term care insurance (LTC). The traditional type of LTC insurance is similar to automobile insurance. You pay a premium and then receive appropriate and needed benefits. These traditional plan premiums do increase with increasing age. Their overall premiums have also been trending upward over time. This type of LTC insurance is optimally purchased during age 50-65. After that, premium increases become unaffordable for most.

LTC insurance is a consideration for most retirement planning. Very wealthy individuals and families may be able to self-insure and not need LTC insurance. Those at the middle income and savings level could be devastated by long-term care expenses and are the most obvious candidates to insure. Those at lowest income and saving level may easily be eligible for Medicaid nursing home benefits and not need LTC insurance.

These traditional long-term care plans usually require a waiting period before benefits kick in, offer a discrete set of benefits and have a limit of delivered benefits. For example, one long-term care plan limits benefits to three years. There is often a premium discount if both spouses enroll together. A hybrid version of long-term care insurance can be linked with a whole-life insurance plan or an annuity. These hybrids have been gaining in popularity, but they do have premiums 2-3x higher than traditional LTC insurance, even for similar benefits. There are also some annuities with long-term care riders.

About 3/4 of Americans over 65 will require long-term care at some point in their lives. Long-term care can range from around $4000/month for home health services or assisted living, to twice that amount for semi-private or private nursing home care. Long-term care insurance will cover care that is either not covered at all, or not the length of time needed, by commercial health insurance or Medicare. Long-term care, when first on the market was affordable and reasonably comprehensive. Now, the combined plans deliver a better value.

HEALTHCARE SPECIALTY SERVICES

SKILLED NURSING & REHABILITATION

Rehabilitation therapy can be done as an outpatient or during an inpatient hospital stay. There are a variety of rehabilitation types. Drug and alcohol rehabilitation are a covered benefit under the Affordable Care Act. The most commonly utilized rehabilitation treatment is nursing home care. Skilling Nursing is the most important. Skilled Nursing Facility care, also called SNF, is almost always in a separate facility from the hospital, serves meals and treatments, and is managed by RNs, LPNs and vocational nurses, under the supervision of a physician. SNFs deliver physical, occupational and speech therapy. There are many SNFs that are part of national corporate chains of facilities. Two thirds of all nursing home patients stay less than 3 months. The majority of patients in nursing homes are over 65. Yet, there is a trend toward fewer people staying in nursing homes per capita.

Individual and group health insurance, including both individual ACA and employer sponsored insurance plans, will vary in their coverage and policies for SNF care. Most of these plans do provide some level and duration of post-acute care in a SNF. These services must be deemed necessary after the hospital stay and are usually just for a short time interval. The SNF will need to be in network for that health plan.

Many individuals and families with no heath or LTC insurance or coverage, or who have exhausted skilled nursing benefits from their insurance, have no other option but to pay nursing home services out of pocket. These payments are often made by liquidating assets, including retirement funds. LTC insurance may pay SNF care, depending on the coverage. Less than 25% of all nursing home patients pay out-of-pocket or LTC insurance. This 25% is desirable for the SNF, since they pay nearly 40% of total nursing home bills. U.S. military veterans may have long-term care benefits from the U.S. Department of Veterans Affairs. Co-pay may be required for some of these Veteran's LTC services.

Skilled nursing care in a SNF is covered under both Medicare and Medicaid. Medicare Part A (Hospital Insurance) covers skilled nursing care provided in a SNF. However, the Medicare member needs to be at inpatient status in a hospital for at least 3 days prior to the transition/transfer to a SNF. Those required 3 days are counted as 3 consecutive midnights in the hospital. They must be bona fide inpatient days, and not observation or days waiting in the ER. The Medicare member can enter the SNF via direct transfer after 3 days in the hospital, or delay SNF admission for up to 30 days upon leaving the hospital after the minimum 3-day stay. The patient can then leave the SNF and reenter the SNF. Or a member can transfer to another SNF. The reentry or transfer needs to occur within 30 days of initial entry. The member would not need another qualifying 3-day inpatient hospital stay to reenter or transfer. The Medicare member's treatment in the SNF can be for the same reason from the prior hospital admission, another reason identified during that same hospital admission or a reason identified while in the SNF. There is no Medicare cost-sharing payment required for the first 20 days in the SNF. Thereafter, the member will have a co-insurance payment for each day from the 21st day until the 100th day. After this 100th day, the Medicare member will have to pay the costs of SNF completely out of pocket.

Medicaid is the shared federal and state funded healthcare program that provides healthcare coverage to low-income residents. Medicaid not only pays for hospital and outpatient care and services, but also pays for home healthcare, hospice care, skilled nursing and long-term nursing home care. The Medicaid nursing home benefit, including the LTC, is referred to as "Institutional Medicaid." Medicaid will pay for long-term nursing home care components, including room and board, nursing care, personal care, and therapy services. Sixty five percent of all U.S. nursing home beds are filled with Medicaid patients. But only 45% of all nursing home bills are paid by Medicaid. Facilities are not eager to give their beds to Medicaid members more cheaply than other payers, and for this reason give them to Medicaid members more sparingly. Medicaid nursing home coverage is allowed if the member requires a nursing home level of care or meets nursing home functional eligibility criteria, and has income and assets below certain state requirements. Each state's criteria for their institutional Medicaid nursing home care may be different. Most states' criteria for medical necessity need for nursing home care relates to the member's level of function, as measured by the need for help with activities of daily living, such as toileting, bathing, and dressing. A Medicaid-qualified nursing home has to be licensed by the state and undergo periodic inspections to meet federal standards. Not all nursing homes accept Medicaid patients or Medicaid payments. Many nursing homes have only a small proportion of beds available for Medicaid patients. This is because Medicaid pays much less for SNF care than other insurances and those paying out of pocket.

The elder law industry was primarily built on helping create a divestment strategy, so that those with favorable resources can otherwise secure Medicaid-funded LTC for a family member. The spouse can then have a comfortable living and the descendent Medicaid member can leave heirs some financial legacy. This is done by the asset transfer through spending down assets. So, this group of attorneys creates a pathway for the more affluent elderly, within the legal frameworks of each state, to move their wealth and transform into or appear more indigent. Then they could qualify for federal/state Medicaid paid LTC for the remainder of their lives. Yet, Medicaid will scrutinize back 5 years from application, to ensure assets or properties were not simply given away, and instead sold or divested for fair market value. Any income generated by the now Medicaid member must be contributed to these LTC or home healthcare services. The Medicaid beneficiary is allowed to keep a small amount of assets as a "personal needs allowance" to pay for uncovered home-based medical expenses, and for food, clothing and housing. The allowance can be used within the nursing home for snacks, subscriptions, and personal products.

Medicaid protects the spouse from becoming destitute, while the other spouse resides in a nursing home. Every state has its own "spousal protection" rules, allowing the home spouse to keep some assets and income to continue living in the community. Medicaid will attempt to recover funds paid, once the Medicaid nursing home beneficiary has died. Medicaid will recover these funds from the estate of the deceased, and therefore called Medicaid "Estate Recovery." The Estate Recovery program began after the passage of the Omnibus Budget Reconciliation Act of 1993 for anyone over age 55 who received Medicaid nursing home, home-based or community services and related hospital and prescription drug services after age 54. Medicaid will not do this if the other spouse is still alive, if there are minor or disabled children involved, or if doing so will cause "undo hardship" to the survivor(s).

References and Links
https://www.medicare.gov/coverage/skilled-nursing-facility-snf-care
https://www.medicaid.gov/medicaid/long-term-services-supports/institutional-long-term-care/nursing-facilities/index.html

HOSPICE

Medicare has established guidelines for hospice admissions, which require a terminal illness in which death is anticipated within six months. This Medicare definition for the need of hospice, is shared and used widely within government and private insurance programs.

Hospice care is delivered by healthcare and community professionals, spiritual leaders and dedicated volunteers. Palliative care is often used interchangeably with hospice, but tends to describe comfort measures used while awaiting a cure. Hospice relates to comfort measures, especially pain control, for those no longer receiving treatment or without an anticipated cure. Hospice can be delivered in hospital wards, free-standing hospice facilities, nursing homes or at one's own home.

The most common terminal diseases that warrant hospice care are Advanced End Stage Senescence or Debility, Amyotrophic Lateral Sclerosis (ALS), liver disease, pulmonary disease such as advanced COPD, dementia, Adult Failure to Thrive, HIV, cancer, stroke and coma. The costs for patients placed in hospice care are paid by Medicare, Medicaid, private insurance, charities or out-of-pocket spending.

Over 40% percent of terminally ill Americans receive hospice care. The majority of hospice care is covered by governmental Medicare, Medicaid, Veterans Administration (VA) and the Department of Defense (DoD). Medicare pays for over 85% of those under hospice care in the US. Medicaid and private insurance contribute another 5-7% of total costs.

Medicare pays for hospice care through Parts A and B, as long as the member is at least 65, has a serious illness, foregoes lifesaving or curative measures and is certified by a doctor to have up to six months to live. Under Medicare, this six-month hospice time allowance can be on a rolling basis with one or more six-month intervals re-certified as appropriate to the diagnosis and prognosis. Therefore, Medicare then initiates hospice care for two 90-day periods in hospice, followed by an unlimited number of 60-day periods. A doctor must re-certify that the patient has six months or less to live, for each period.

Medicare will cover a range of hospice services, including nursing and doctor care, social work and counseling, occupational and speech therapies, medical appliances and supplies, as well as bereavement counseling for the family members. Medicare also offers Respite Care, so that the hospice patient can stay for up to five days in a Medicare-approved nursing home, hospital or hospice facility in order to give the family care-givers their own break from caregiving. Medicare will not cover room and board, ambulance or emergency room costs or any treatment or pharmaceuticals that intend to cure illness.

End-of-life hospice care is offered to children with disabilities or adults who meet Medicaid's financial eligibility criteria. Medicaid hospice eligibility requirements are identical to those of Medicare. Yet, Medicaid hospice coverage can vary from state to state. Those dual eligible for both Medicare and Medicaid can have uncovered Medicare hospice costs paid by Medicaid. These Medicare-uncovered, Medicaid-covered hospice expenses would include outpatient prescription drugs and LTC. This important distinction of Medicaid, not seen with Medicare benefits, is that the former will pay at least 95% of room and board costs for hospice patients in a nursing home.

Active military and its retirees and dependents receive hospice care through TRICARE. The VA sponsored Civilian Health and Medical Program of the Department of Veterans Affairs delivers hospice coverage for those eligible beneficiaries of certain deceased or disabled veterans. Private health insurance plans vary widely in terms of coverage. Some may have limits on hospice expenses. However, most private insurers do cover hospice costs since it is cheaper than acute end-of-life hospital costs. Those without governmental or private insurance access to hospice care, will either pay out of pocket, oftentimes through a sliding scale, or fortunately be assisted by a charitable organization.

References and Links
https://www.medicare.gov/coverage/hospice-care
https://www.medicaid.gov/medicaid/benefits/hospice-benefits/index.html
https://hospicefoundation.org/Hospice-Care/Hospice-Services

AUTOPSY

An autopsy is the examination of the dead body, the tissues and internal organs and evaluates the character and chemistries of the blood and other body fluids. An autopsy can be requested by the doctor, the family next of kin or the state's medical examiner or coroner. An autopsy is done by a pathologist, in most states. It is usually done when the circumstances of death are suspicious or unknown. Essentially, all states request an autopsy when someone dies in a suspicious, unusual, or unnatural way. Some states require an autopsy when death occurs outside the presence of a doctor. This can be a death at home, work or on the street. Over half of the states require an autopsy when the cause of death could be from a public health threat. This would be suspected food poisoning or rapidly spreading infection.

Some private pathology services will do an autopsy for a fee. A private autopsy can be done if the death occurred outside the jurisdiction of a medical examiner. It can also be considered if there was suspected malpractice, for insurance reasons, a potential health risk to the family or as a second opinion from a previous autopsy. Neither private insurance, nor Medicare or Medicaid, will pay for a private autopsy. It is paid out of pocket or as part of a litigation expense.

There are some certain religious concerns against autopsies, in order to keep the deceased's body whole and undisturbed or the need to not delay burial. Medical examiners, under these circumstances, may expedite or respectfully modify how the autopsy is done. Yet, even under these religious constraints, states will mandate any autopsy in order to investigate a crime or control a public health threat.

TRANSPLANTATION

Over 100,000 prospective organ recipients in this country, are waiting for an organ match. These are many more waiting, than organs available. The kidney is the most often transplanted organ. This is because the harvested kidney can come from either living or deceased donors. We have two kidneys, and a donor can easily live, with one kidney. Other organs regularly transplanted come from deceased organ donors. These are liver, lungs, heart, pancreas, and intestines. Hands and faces were added to the organ transplant list within the last few years. Yet, living donation can also come from one lung, or a portion of the liver, pancreas, or intestine.

Human tissues can be donated within 24 hours of death, and placed into tissue banks, even for prolonged periods of time. These banked tissue donations include corneas, middle ear, skin, heart valves, bone, veins, cartilage, tendons, and ligaments. These donated tissues can restore sight, cover burns, repair hearts or veins, and damaged connective tissue and cartilage. Healthy adults can donate blood stem cells to be used in stem cell transplants. Stem cells can also be donated from umbilical cord blood. Blood and platelets donations, as are commonly done in all communities through such events as blood drives and plasma clinics, can occur every 56 days and every four weeks, respectively.

Each transplant program, which are usually associated with a medical school university, college or large advanced medical center, has oversight in terms of who they will accept for transplantation into their program. Once accepted for a transplant, that program will put you on the national "waitlist." The United Network for Organ Sharing (UNOS) manages the waiting lists for all transplant programs. UNOS matches donors to recipients. The wait for an organ can be days or years. Donor and recipient compatibility matching occur by creating a smaller list from the larger wait list. This smaller list is based on the organ's allocation policy which includes geographic region, genetic compatibility, condition of the organ, and the recipient's disease severity, along with the recipient's time waiting.

Transplant costs are funded by private or government insurance and out-of-pocket spending. Costs or also supplemented by funding of several transplant organizations. Complete costs for transplantation include the donated organ transportation and recipient transplant surgery or transplant procedure, post-transplant care, including immunosuppressive medications, and any transplant or immunosuppression complications that may occur. Related transplantation expenses include all needed travel and lodging related to the impending or completed transplant.

Many insurance companies offer variable coverage for transplant costs. Some allow costs up to a maximum spend. Many insurance policies will not cover any transplants or procedures considered experimental or investigational (EI). Appeal to the health plan is always available, to challenge denied coverage for a transplant service. Medicare Parts A and B will cover transplantation and its care, including immunosuppression for heart, lung, kidney, pancreas, intestine, and liver organ transplants. Most Medicaid programs cover transplants performed in that state, unless there are no centers in your region. For which, that state Medicaid will cover costs in another state. Government funding for families of active-duty, retired, or deceased military personnel may be available through TRICARE. TRICARE covers living donor kidney, liver, and lung transplants. Transplantation is an exciting and growing option for many patients with end-stage organ disease or dysfunction, deformities or injuries and for the rejuvenation of aged tissues. Transplantation is expensive and sometimes fraught with challenges, but can often be the last hope for many waiting.

References and Links
https://unos.org/
https://www.medicare.gov/coverage/organ-transplants

TELEHEALTH

Telehealth is the use of electronic, digital and other means of information and communication technologies to access health information and manage healthcare. Computers and ubiquitous mobiles devices (cell phones, tablets) are usually the main platforms for this communication. During these telemedical communications, the interaction is therefore between the provider, often a doctor, and the patient. Telemedicine was once a slowly developing branch of medicine, primarily due to little or no reimbursement. It has since exploded since the COVID-19 pandemic. Reimbursement therefore was implements or increased, due to this event.

Telehealth is broadly considered anything from direct doctor-patient interactions to internet searching for healthcare and disease process information. Ideally, the internet searching leads to reputable websites. The University of Michigan has put together their list of quality health websites at https://uhs.umich.edu/websites. Telehealth can even include the use of exercise, diet and health applications on a cellular phone. Telehealth can be the access to patient's electronic medical records (EMR), sometimes called patient portals, in order to review lab results, upcoming appointments, review previous office notes, refill prescriptions and communicate with your providers. Telehealth can be remote monitoring of heart rate and rhythm, blood pressure, blood glucose, sleep patterns and even accidental falls. The personal health record is also part of the spectrum of telehealth. These personal health records are stand-alone patient consolidated health information, aggregated into an electronic protected form.

The most important component of telehealth is telemedicine or the virtual appointment. This is when the patient electronically meets with the provider for an office appointment. This can be a synchronous real-time telephone call or live audio-video interaction, typically with a patient using a smartphone, tablet, or computer. The virtual appointment proceeds as any other office-based face-to-face appointment, beginning with the discussion of the problem and review of other medical history. The physical examination can be done by the provider's observation, the patient's interactions with diagnostic devices or tests, or an assistant or nurse on-site with the patient. These digital examinations can include digital stethoscopes, otoscopes and ultrasound devices.

It is becoming vital that both patient and provider have health plan access and reimbursement for telemedicine. Insurance payers and medical professional associations had supported the transition to telehealth services during the COVID-19 pandemic. The Health and Human Services Office for Civil Rights issued guidance loosening restrictions of HIPAA-covered healthcare providers who, in good faith, provide telehealth services to patients using remote communication technologies, including FaceTime, Facebook Messenger, Google Hangouts, Zoom, or Skype. But, these telehealth interactions are forbidden from using less secure public-facing platforms, such as Facebook Live, Twitch, and TikTok.

CMS issued multiple waivers for telehealth during the COVID-19 pandemic. Medicare Part B (Medical Insurance) therefore covers certain telehealth services. Co-pays and deductibles still do apply. The Medicare member will pay the same as in-person services. Some Medicare Advantage plans may pay even more for telehealth than traditional Medicare.

Medicaid programs that are administered by the states can choose whether or not to cover telehealth services. Many states including California, Colorado, Texas, Mississippi and the District of Colombia do cover telehealth in their Medicaid programs. Very few private health plans had covered any degree of telehealth over the last 5-10 years. Yet, all major private health insurers began covering telehealth during the COVID-19 pandemic. The pandemic changed quite a few ways of doing business. More worked remotely. Less traveled for business by airplane. It is expected that these trends will continue through and after recovery. Same with telehealth. It is expected that telehealth services will continue, as reimbursable services, as part of our integral healthcare, into the future

Telehealth functions effectively, in most situations, analogous to in-person evaluations. Telehealth does have some limitations. Telehealth usually cannot cross state borders, unless the provider is licensed in the other patient's state. Some patients have limited access to telehealth technologies. There are some

American households without internet. Some patients are unable to understand and engage in the telehealth technologies. Finally, there are some important or urgent health conditions which are still best served with an in-person evaluation. Telehealth has been stubborn to take hold, even as secure technologies entered the market place. The main holdup was reimbursement; that has changed. Telehealth has been meeting these challenges and well on the way toward accessing our healthcare.

References and Links
https://www.hhs.gov/coronavirus/telehealth/index.html
https://www.ama-assn.org/practice-management/digital/5-huge-ways-pandemic-has-changed-telemedicine

EMERGENCY ROOM

One goes to the Emergency Room (ER) when experiencing a severe injury or concerning symptoms, or a disorder that requires a high level of care. A few common examples of medical conditions that bring patients to an ER include chest pain, severe-onset headache or car accident with loss of consciousness. The ER is also a place where people go for simple sniffles and sneezes. Unfortunately, the ER is the place where indigent and those with no insurance, often go simply for primary care. A small proportion of Medicaid and Medicare members use ER resources at a higher level compared to the remaining majority. ER evaluation and care of significant illness or injuries, can lead directly to hospital admission.

The free-standing ER can be affiliated with a hospital, or a hospital can have its own imbedded ER. An ER can also be free-standing and independent. The quality of care and acuity and severity of incoming patients into the independent free-standing ER are the same as in the hospital-based ER. The free-standing ER will have high-technology imaging and will do some medical interventions. The free-standing ER can set fractures, suture lacerations and drain abscesses. They may also treat some degree of trauma. Free-standing ERs will need to transport more severe and acute conditions, such as heart attack, stroke and unstable injuries, to the hospital-based ER for immediate interventional treatments.

References and Links

https://www.hcup-us.ahrq.gov/reports/statbriefs/sb221-Super-Utilizer-ED-Visits-Payer-2014.jsp
https://www.acep.org/patient-care/policy-statements/freestanding-emergency-departments/

TRAUMA CENTERS

Hospitals are tertiary and quaternary care centers with specialized expertise and equipment that accept injured in various capacities and can care for severe levels of illnesses. Hospitals also accept trauma based on their level of capabilities. The American College of Surgeons (ACS) designates hospitals as trauma center levels I through V. The ACS also administers the Advanced Trauma Life Support (ATLS) training for both residents and attending physicians. ATLS certification has a 4-year duration, until recertification. The ATLS focuses on traumatic injuries, such as broken bones and penetrating injuries. While the American Heart Association certifies healthcare providers and others who care for patients to mitigate and treat acute heart conditions, such as heart attack. These certifications are either Basic Life Support (BCLS) or the more Advanced Cardiac Life Support (ACLS). The latter is mostly administered during cardiac events in the hospitals or clinics. These include CPR, chest compressions (cardiopulmonary resuscitation), defibrillation and at times, administration of heart medications.

The ACS Level I Trauma Centers accept the highest volume of the most severely injured. These Level I Trauma Centers must have surgeons, anesthesiologists and other specialists in-house 24 hours and be an accepting referral for the neighboring communities' facilities and providers. In comparison, the Level V Trauma Center is the lowest designation. Level V will only have a basic ER that may not be staffed with 24/7 ATLS trained Physicians and Nurses. These Level Vs are more often the small and rural hospitals. The Level V Center will transfer the severest patients to Level I - III Trauma Centers. Either by ground transportation or helicopter.

References and Links
https://www.facs.org/Quality-Programs/Trauma/ATLS
https://cpr.heart.org/en/cpr-courses-and-kits/healthcare-professional/acls

URGENT CARE & RETAIL CLINICS

Urgent care clinics are used for more minor healthcare complaints and conditions. They are also used by patients who either have to pay out of pocket or have a higher cost sharing health insurance, to otherwise used a traditional ER. Urgent care clinics usually have shorter wait times to see a provider, compared to the traditional ER. Urgent care clinics may not be staffed 24 hours/7 days weeks, like a traditional ER; but they are often open on weekends and weekday evenings. These clinics can have weakened continuity of care with the primary physicians, since they are not often affiliated with those providers through an electronic medical record or connect by phone follow-up. These clinics may have inadequate discharge planning.

Some chain drugstores and even big box stores with pharmacies (such as Walmart), are opening embedded retail health clinics. These retail health clinics function as a hybrid between a primary care office and urgent care clinic. They see patients with minor injuries, do sports exams for children and vaccinations for anyone.

One is always best served to determine whether the urgent care or retail clinic is considered in network or out of network, for their health plan. Some insurers will pay in-network costs for any emergency care. But any deemed out-of-network care will have higher cost sharing.

OBSERVATION

A patient may come to a hospital-based ER with a complaint, such as chest pain, and then undergo medical evaluation. But, can be other illnesses or injuries. That evaluation may not identify a problem that would require immediate intervention or admission into a hospital bed. As in our heart pain example, maybe the pain lessened and the laboratory blood enzymes and stress testing were not conclusive. This patient may be placed in "observation" while monitored by a nurse until stable or angina is ruled out. Once stable, this patient would be discharged. The discharge is from the temporary observation and not from a formal hospital admission. This distinction is vital.

The observation may be in a separate outpatient unit or even in a hospital bed, but without being designated as formally admitted to the hospital. So, on its face, the observation may even look like a hospital admission. In contradistinction, formal hospital admission is what defines inpatient status. These differences illustrated are essentially important because the commercial health plan or Medicare will pay for your hospital observation stay as a lower-cost outpatient service. Those observation days and services will be paid less than if delivered as an inpatient.

This situation becomes even more troublesome when someone is in observation for days and then requires transfer to a skilled-nursing facility for further recuperation or therapies. This SNF transfer and subsequent SNF services would only be covered under Medicare if the patient as an inpatient for at least 3 days. Observation days do not count toward this 3-day Medicare requirement. Unfortunately, this has become a common, confusing and frustrating situation for patients and families.

The 3-day inpatient rule has been waived, at the SNFs discretion, during the COVID pandemic. This waiver will expire April 21,2021.

References and Links
https://www.medicare.gov/what-medicare-covers/what-part-a-covers/inpatient-or-outpatient-hospital-status
https://www.cms.gov/Outreach-and-Education/Medicare-Learning-Network-MLN/MLNProducts/Downloads/SNF3DayRule-MLN9730256.pdf
https://www.medicare.gov/what-medicare-covers/what-part-a-covers/inpatient-or-outpatient-hospital-status

COMPLEMENTARY & ALTERNATIVE MEDICINE

Complementary Medicine, in other words alternatives to the traditional western scientific model-based standards medicine, has been gaining access and influence in this country. This is due to the melting pot society with increased acceptance and practice of other cultures, especially in this respect, Eastern medical practices. This is particularly true of the inquiry and adoption of some Chinese practices of medicine. These being acupuncture and herb medicine.

Complementary medicine is also called "integrative," in that it integrates alternative therapies with the western scientific treatment strategies. There are hundreds of alternative treatments, some effective and others not effective. Some are even injurious and dangerous. A macrobiotic can be used to replace a deficiency. But its overuse, which sometimes occurred during its fad popularity, can cause some to take in excess. The fat-soluble vitamins, A, D, E and K, are not easily excreted in urine like the water-soluble vitamins. Mega-doses fat soluble vitamins excess can lead to toxicities. Melatonin is widely suggested for insomnia. There are number of vitamins, minerals and herbs, that are increasing used for certain ailments, conditions or emotional states. Few with any scientific basis.

Yet, there are have been considerable new and novel health ideas that have led to improved lives and lifestyles. Neighborhood jogging became popular in the 1960s and has led to more of the population getting outside and walking, running or bike-riding today, all activities that improve health and well-being. Kids these days would benefit from less computer screen time and more breeze, forest and wildlife.

There are a variety of these complementary methods. Some are as old as civilization, while others are a recent development, or variations on older treatments. More noted and accepted alternatives include acupuncture, homeopathy, naturopathy and Chinese medicine and pharmaceuticals. Healing of the body by touch includes western versions of chiropractic and osteopathic techniques, as well as eastern influenced massage, tai chi, yoga and other body movements therapies. Other alternatives are treating the mind-body connection with meditation, biofeedback and hypnosis. Or using the senses to heal, such as with art or music therapy or the use of imagery.

Three alternative treatments show clear confidence in health benefits. These are eastern acupuncture, music and animal therapies. Any treatment must consider results not related to the treatment itself. This refers to the placebo effect. Other non-medical forces and environments confound healing in either positive or negative ways. The placebo effect is essentially getting something for nothing. The best scientific medical studies evaluate a legitimate promising treatment arm that is compared to a control or "sham" arm. This control arm can be a placebo, something like a sugar pill or something without pharmaceutic properties. This experimental drug response is then compared to the control, the placebo effect. The placebo effect is improvement expected from the going through the motions of treatment, but without receiving the real active treatment. This placebo effect is seen in 15% and up to 50% of cases. One needs to always consider if an alternative has a scientific basis for effect or is disguised as a placebo effect or an effect from other confounding interacting variables. Nevertheless, placebo effect that leads to healing, is a part of both effective and ineffective treatments, Western and Eastern treatments.

Each heath plan may differ on the coverage of complementary or alternative treatments. Most insurers, usually the larger plans, will cover chiropractic and acupuncture. The vast majority of other alternative treatments may be uncovered by health plans. The health plan beneficiary may therefore decide to engage in the alternative treatment and pay out of pocket. Medicare will generally not cover what is considered alternative or complementary medicine. They will cover chiropractic treatment to correct spinal subluxation, some nutrition therapy and smoking-cessation counseling. Medicare now covers 12 acupuncture sessions within a 90-day period, and up to 20 sessions a year, to treat chronic lower back pain. Music therapy is not reimbursed directly but may be covered by Medicare as part of a package of treatment within SNF, rehabilitation, psychiatric or hospice services. Medicare does not cover massage, Reiki, Rolfing and trigger point therapy. Nor does Medicare cover naturopathy or homeopathy. The American medical community has been slow and prudent in the adoption of alternative healthcare treatments, but maintains an open mind with current acceptance of some forms and going forward.

References and Links
https://www.nccih.nih.gov/health/complementary-alternative-or-integrative-health-whats-in-a-name
https://www.medicareadvantage.com/coverage/does-medicare-cover-holistic-medicine

SUPPLEMENTAL INSURANCE

DENTAL

There was once a time when there was only one or two dental insurance plans available. These were primarily as an individual or family benefit of employment. Now, dentists are less interested in family dentistry, preferring to branch into cosmetic dentistry and implants. With this trend, less dentists today are in-network for the array of dental plans currently available. Beyond dentists, there are oral surgeons who undergo medical training and handle tooth extractions, gum procedures and round through hospitals. Some office oral surgeon services, and always those rendered to hospital inpatients, are reimbursed by the medical insurance plan. The dental plans today vary by provider structure, provider accessibility as network, coverage, fees, cost sharing and maximum charges.

These dental plans can be what we think of as traditional indemnity that allows any dentist to charge "usual, customary and reasonable" (UCR) fees, up to an annual beneficiary allowance. These indemnity dental plans are often Preferred Provider Organizations (PPO) of network dentists that accept the maximum allowable fees for delivered services. A more restrictive version of the PPO, is Exclusive Provider Organizations (EPO), which requires care by an even smaller group of participating dentists. The Dental Health Maintenance Organizations (DHMO), often functioning through capitation, pay the dentists monthly per members and require the delivery of contracted services at no cost or reduced cost to those members. The member can seek out-of-network care, but at a lower reimbursement. Another variation of this is the Table or Schedule of Allowances dental plans which are indemnities that pay set rates for dental procedures and require the member to pay the balance.

The dental fees can be paid through direct out-of-pocket patient reimbursement. This can be done by paying the stated dental fees or negotiating down these fees, either before or after the dental services. There is a Direct Reimbursement type of dental plan that is self-funded, allowing the member to go to a dentist of their choice, pay that dentist directly and then seek reimbursement. Often these are set-dollar-amount plans. Finally, there are a few Discount or Referral schemes, which are gaining in popularity with employers, from companies contracting discounted fees for dental services.

Most dental plans cover preventative and basic restorative dental services, including fillings and extractions. Higher premium "full coverage" dental plans will include these coverage features, along with major restorative services, such as bridges, crowns, dentures and orthodontia. About half of all American adults have dental insurance. Of those, 1/4 do not use dental services during that year of coverage. Dental fees have increased 20% in the last decade. Many people, especially during times of low economic activity, defer getting needed dental services.

There is no Cadillac dental plan. Nearly all dental insurance will have some exclusions and limitations on spend and include an annual maximum. The maximum spend amount can be across all types of dental services or as individual limits for each individual service. The member bears the cost of all dental services, after surpassing these insurance maximums. Since this is annual, the spending limits do reset on the dental insurance renewal anniversary. Only dental HMOs and discounted dental plans will technically have no annual maximum. But these are limited to preventive and basic restorative services and include cost sharing for these dental services.

Examination of the highest-level full coverage individual dental plans available to the public could not identify one without an annual maximum. For example, United Healthcare Dental Premium Elite has a $1500 annual benefit limit after 4 years of subscription. Likewise, Delta Dental PPO, which also offers dental plans on the ACA exchange, has an annual $1500 maximum. Spirit Dental has a plan with a $5000 annual maximum.

Dental services through dental insurance plans can require a co-payment and annual deductible. The dental office may submit your dental services claim. If not, the member will have to submit the claim to the dental insurer, in order to get reimbursement. Most preventative care, such as teeth cleaning, x-rays and evaluations, will not require cost sharing. Some dental insurance plans have a waiting period for major work which may have been needed and delayed, before the time of current insurance subscription. Dental implants are not usually covered on standard dental insurance plans. Many insurance plans do allow implant benefits to be bought and added to their plans. Cosmetic and orthodontics are almost never part of a standard dental insurance plan.

Dental plans used to be straightforward, were accepted by local dentists widely and covered most services with cost sharing. Today, there is a dizzying array of dental insurance and reimbursement products. There are more products with less enthusiasm from the actual practitioners. The need and type of dental insurance should be weighed against the ability or willingness to negotiate dental work as you go.

References and Links
https://success.ada.org/en/dental-benefits/dental-plan-overview

VISION

Vision insurance is mostly offered by employers as an elective insurance product to their employees. Few buy on the individual market. Some vision insurance plans charge an initial enrollment fee. The employee can enroll once each year, during the company's open-enrollment period. Monthly premiums are usually between $5 and $15 per person, excluding co-pays or deductibles. Vision insurance as the cost of the monthly premium, reduces the costs of glasses, contacts, and eye exams. The least expensive plans may only cover glasses, and not contact lenses. This insurance can often offset the cost of LASIK.

These vision insurance plans vary as to coverage and costs covered for annual exams, glasses and contact lenses. A co-payment cost sharing will be required if the vision insurer does not offer full coverage for goods and services. These insurance plans often require purchasing vision exams and products at certain network providers or stores. They may also require purchasing of certain brands and could have price limits on these goods. LASIK is almost never fully covered through these vision plans. Eye surgeries and treatments for conditions like glaucoma and cataracts will not be covered on vision insurance and instead covered through medical insurance.

Seventy percent of the U.S. population wears glasses or contacts. Vision insurance may save an individual $100 each year with an annual eye exam and purchase of glasses, when compared to out-of-pocket payments. But there is an equally high likelihood of net financial loss by paying premium for unused benefits. Out-of-pocket purchases for vision goods and services may be below the annual payout under a vision plan.

The value of vision insurance is widely argued. An eye exam can be found, at big box or other retailers, for $50-60. Chain eyewear stores will regularly have promotions and discounts for glasses. Many eyeglass high-volume web-based companies have increased the ease and dramatically lowered the costs for eyeglass purchases. One is served best to make these calculations of expected vision-related expenditures for the coming year, in order to determine if buying vision insurance will lead to cost savings.

References and Links
https://finance.zacks.com/worth-taking-vision-insurance-10006.html

ACCIDENTAL

Accident insurance helps pay out-of-pocket costs from an accident or injury. Accidental injury would be an unforeseen and unfortunate mishap, including falls, cuts, burns, road accidents, bites, stings and drowning. Accident insurers may or may not include risky (e.g., skydiving) or self-inflicted injuries. This insurance is supplemental to your medical insurance and provides lump-sum cash payments directly to you, as indemnity.

Accident insurance is complementary and not a replacement for medical insurance. Medical health insurance covers hospital and doctor expenses for illness or injury. Accident insurance intends to supplement this medical insurance coverage but with low-priced premiums and narrowly defined coverage. An accident rider can sometimes be purchased with medical insurance plans. Life insurance can overlap some coverage in the event of accidental death. Life insurance is financial protection with payouts to the survivors. An accident policy will similarly pay out a described sum to the named beneficiary, in the event of the subscriber's death. Yet, accident insurance will not pay out for death from natural causes or illnesses. There is also some overlap with disability insurance. A disability from an accidental injury will receive an accident insurance payout up to a specific percentage of the insured sum.

Accident insurance is secondary to medical health insurance. Accident insurance does not directly reimburse your doctors and hospitals. Instead they pay out directly to the beneficiary based on a schedule of events. Out-of-pocket costs that get paid through accident insurance include emergency treatment, hospital stays, and medical examinations, services and goods, as well as transportation and lodging needs.

Most accident insurance is offered as an option during an employer's open enrollment period. It is not often sought by consumers in the open individual or family insurance market. It may be considered more often by those healthcare conservative individuals who prefer to be over-insured. Accident insurance may benefit those with high deductible medical insurance, since it can be used for related healthcare or any unrelated costs or savings. Most Americans are satisfied with their healthcare, life, and disability insurance coverages in the event of an accidental event.

References and Links
https://www.coverage.com/insurance/auto/accident-insurance/

CANCER

The American Cancer Society estimates that 1.8 million Americans will be diagnosed with cancer this year. More than 600,000 Americans die from cancer each year. One half of all men and 1/3 of all women will be diagnosed with cancer during their lifetime. Cancer insurance provides financial protection for a cancer-related healthcare event, as a supplement to medical insurance. It would also supplement coverage and benefits for cancer-related disability and death, from those found in disability and life insurance plans. Cash benefits can be used for cancer-related healthcare costs or even to pay the mortgage and utility bills. Cancer insurance is secondary to other insurance payouts.

Like all insurances, cancer insurance will vary by cost and coverage. Cancer insurance requires a monthly premium and pays out in lump sum, just like accident insurance. Those cash payments vary according to the insured event. Some of these cancer insurance plans cover preventive care, heart attack and stroke, and experimental cancer treatments.

Most will only insure adults and some plans terminate coverage at age 64-65. Others allow coverage, but with reduced benefits after age 70. Some exclude pre-existing conditions, have a waiting period between events and/or have a waiting period before any coverage and payout. Cancer insurance could be considered in those individuals that desire the comfort of robust insuring, have a high risk of cancer in the family or have a high-deductible health plan.

<u>References and Links</u>
https://www.cancer.org/treatment/finding-and-paying-for-treatment/understanding-health-insurance.html

PHARMACEUTICALS

RESEARCH & DEVELOPMENT (R&D)

It takes up to 15 years, at a cost of $2.6 billion, to bring a new prescription drug to the market. Each successful drug developed on that prototype may cost hundreds of millions of dollars. Many drug prototypes are explored, often even hundreds, before an effective new drug candidate is fully developed. Only one in 10 new drugs that enter into clinical trials eventually gets Federal Drug Administration (FDA) approval. Only 5% of the over 7,000 rare diseases have current drug treatment.

There is no doubt that pharmaceuticals do give us high social value in the improvement of health and longevity. Yet, this is at a great cost. It is often believed that this cost may be too high. There is evidence that higher profits do lead to greater research and development (R&D). This occurs only up to a point. There is a diminishing return to the consumer, with increasing pharmaceutical companies' revenues.

Drug development as outlined by the FDA required processes, can be reflected in five stages. First, the discovery and development of a new drug begins with basic laboratory evaluations. Often, this is done examining many, sometimes hundreds, of molecules and compounds. Next comes further laboratory and animal research in order to answer basic questions of the elected drug's safety and viability. Clinical research follows, using human subjects to again test for safety and efficacy. At completion, the FDA reviews all of this information and makes a determination to approve the drug, or not. The FDA continues to monitor the safety of this approved drug after it has been released for public use.

The FDA clinical research protocol is very stringent, involving 4 phases. Twenty to 100 volunteers of people with the studied disease are recruited and treated over several months in order to determine dosage and confirm safety. Nearly 3/4 of Phase 1 drugs go to the next stage. Phase 2 involves use in several hundred people, to determine efficacy and any side effects. Phase 2 lasts up to two years. One third of drugs move from Phase 2 to Phase 3. This next phase continues to examine adverse effects, by increasing the number disease-related volunteers up to 3,000 and lasting up to 4 more years. About 1/4 of drugs survive these three phases, into Phase 4. The final phase is completed with several thousand more volunteers to confirm safety and efficacy. Success in Phase 4 leads to allowing the drug to enter the marketplace.

There are several considerations to control drug costs. These include decreasing the time interval that drugs are protected and solely produced by that manufacturer, including the speedier introduction of generics, as well as cost controls. R&D is both costly and risky. The cost of producing more of the same drugs already in the market, is extremely cheap. The cost of imitating a current drug is also very low. There is some lower level "differentiated" product competition between patented drugs that treat the same disease. But this doesn't tend to nudge the prices down much.

Overall the price that can be attained for a new drug will influence the amount of R&D funds put into it. More R&D funds will be placed into the development of a novel drug that treat a large population. Less funds will be used to treat rare diseases or where similar drugs are already near or in the marketplace. It is anticipated that there is some restraint on sales of a new drug, as prices increase. This is more aligned with the importance of the disease being treated, relative to its costs. Yet, health insurance pays a substantial portion of prescription costs. The health plan will pay all, even for approved hyper-expensive drugs, once the out-of-pocket maximum has been met. Sometimes drug developers can show that the high cost of one or several treatments outweigh the overall treatment costs of the untreated disease. So, much of the constraints are within the health plan utilization review of that emerging drug or their delegated pharmacy benefit mangers (PBM).

References and Links
https://www.fda.gov/drugs/development-approval-process-drugs

GENERICS

A generic drug according to the FDA is biologically the same as the original drug. The original drug is also called a pioneer, or reference drug, which is usually a branded drug. The generic and original drugs are therefore identical in dosage, form, absorption, route of administration, strength, quality, safety, and performance. In other words, the generic will be of the same bio-equivalence as the original. The generic drug should also have the same intended uses as the original. The generic will meet the same batch requirements and will be manufactured according to the same Good Manufacturing Practice regulations, required by the FDA.

Generics encompass nearly 90% of all prescription drugs in this country today. There is significant healthcare costs savings with the use of generics. Generics are only 26% of all prescription costs. Side-by-side, generic medications cost 13% compared with their branded counterparts. Generics have also led to improvements in indirect healthcare costs such as therapy adherence and compliance. One tends to take the prescription drug when the drug treatment is affordable. Generics save Americans nearly $300 billion a year in healthcare costs. But it wasn't always this way.

Congress passed the Federal Food, Drug, and Cosmetic Act (FDCA) of 1938 in response to the deaths of over 100 people taking an Elixir Sulfanilamide. Elixir Sulfanilamide was produced by the S.E. Massengill Company of Bristol, Tennessee, and contained toxic ethylene glycol which tragically led to kidney failure and, in this case, mass death. During this era, there were no animal testing or other premarket safety regulations in place before introducing new drugs. The FDCA required all drugs introduced after this 1938 incident to be proven safe through manufacturer testing and FDA clearance before marketing.

The safety requirement was strengthened again in 1962 through the Kefauver-Harris Drug Amendments. If the pioneer drug, even back to 1938, was found unsafe, then that drug and all the copies that followed were removed. Thereafter, the FDA allowed proof of safety and efficacy through a scientific literature-based New Drug Application. The Hatch-Waxman Act of 1984, also called Drug Price Competition and Patent Term Restoration Act, expedited generics into the market without the requirement to repeat efficacy and safety research, but only if the reference versions were released after 1962. This legislation did protect the branded drug by extending their patent protection for up to 5 years. The patent extension was increased to 20 years after original filing, through the 1994 Uruguay Rounds Agreements Act. The Generic Drug Enforcement Act of 1992 required generic drug manufacturers to include more scientific data concerning quality and bio-equivalence.

American consumers, either as health plan beneficiaries or direct purchasers, are the major drivers of generic drug sales. Federal and state health plans, as original supporters of generic programs, have become major purchasers of generics. Doctors and pharmacies originally were more opposed to generics, ("dispense as written") but now are aligned and advocate to serve the needs of their patients.

References and Links
https://www.fda.gov/drugs/buying-using-medicine-safely/generic-drugs
https://www.fda.gov/regulatory-information/laws-enforced-fda

BIOLOGICALS

Biologicals, also called biological therapeutics or biological medications are grown and purified from cells of bacteria, yeast, plant or animal cells to create a group of widely used medications. They are made from the entire cell or tissue or parts of those cells, such as sugars, proteins, or DNA. Biologicals are immune modulators, monoclonal antibodies, growth factors and products that are more commonly recognized, such as vaccines, human blood and plasma. Some are even tissues for transfer. They are complex mixtures, often coming from diverse sources, that are not easily identified or characterized.

Biologicals differ from what we consider typical prescribed medications. The former are purified proteins made from living cultures and blood, while common prescription drugs are synthetically made small molecules. Biologicals also differ as being less stable than the typical prescription drug. They are heat-sensitive and require clean handling and administration. Biologicals may even be produced through biotechnology and other emerging methods. These biologicals are highly regulated and tested, at each level, to ensure consistency across all batches, manufacturers and countries of production. They often treat illness when there is no other option or method of treatment.

Humira (adalimumab) is a common example of a biological. It is used to treat rheumatoid arthritis, psoriasis and Crohn's disease. It is a monoclonal antibody which works by trapping molecules, called antigens. In this way it decreases the inflammation associated with these diseases.

Botox (onabotulinumtoxinA) is another well recognized biological. Botox is extracted from the paralyzing bacteria called Clostridium botulinum. In nature this bacterium produces a powerful paralyzing toxin. It was initially pioneered to inhibit eyelid twitching and release tightening of the muscle band between the esophagus and stomach. It is more famously used to flatten aging wrinkles on the face. It is also used to treat excessive underarm sweating, migraines and loss of bladder control from spinal cord disease or injury.

Biologicals are an increasing area of research and utilization. The complexities in processing and use translate into higher costs. Pharmaceuticals, especially biologicals have become the costliest component of modern healthcare. Yet, they are essential in treating and curing some serious diseases.

References and Links

https://www.who.int/health-topics/biologicals#tab=tab_1

https://www.fda.gov/about-fda/fda-organization/center-biologics-evaluation-and-research-cber

https://www.humira.com/

https://www.botox.com/

HEALTHCARE OUTSIDE THE U.S.

VACATIONING
INTERNATIONAL
COVERAGE

The U.S. State Department warns that domestic health insurance coverage does not extend to US citizens overseas. This means anywhere outside the U.S.A. The State Department suggests that before any travel, checking with your current health plan to determine if and how it covers you while traveling to other countries. This is important because each plan will either not cover or cover a different set of services at different rates.

It is suggested to purchase supplemental insurance when traveling outside the country. There are more than a dozen of these services, including such companies as Allianz. This supplemental travel insurance should include routine services, emergency services, emergency transportation and evacuation and cancelation insurance. The State Department will help distraught U.S. travelers when requested while overseas, through its U.S. Embassies or Consulates. They will help you locate medical services, inform your friends or family back in the U.S. of your health predicament and assist in the transfer of funds to you, in order to financially support your situation, there.

Many U.S. regulated health plans will pay "customary and reasonable" hospital costs abroad but, you will always pay more. This overseas coverage is generally limited to reimbursement at the higher member cost-sharing out-of-network rates. You will have to pay the foreign hospital or foreign physician services out-of-pocket and then seek reimbursement from your health plan after returning home.

U.S. health plans won't cover overseas prescriptions. Nor will they cover the very high cost of medical evacuation. These plans often will not cover overseas injuries related to terrorist attacks, acts of war, natural disasters, adventure activities such as scuba diving and mountain climbing, and exacerbations of pre-existing conditions. Even a medical "emergency" may be defined differently by different health plans. Most health plans consider "emergency" as real jeopardy to you without immediate medical attention.

With few exceptions, original Medicare (i.e., Part A or B) will not cover medical costs overseas. Traditional Medicare will cover in the U.S. territories of the Virgin Islands, Guam, American Samoa and the North Mariana Islands or on a cruise ship in territorial waters adjoining U.S. territories. Medicare will cover inpatient, doctor, ambulance and dialysis under an emergency and if the foreign care is closer than the nearest U.S. hospital. The foreign hospital is not required to submit claims to Medicare. You will have to pay the overseas provider or facility and then submit your claims back in the U.S. to Medicare. Medicare Advantage plans may differ from traditional Medicare overseas, and follow coverage similar to their commercial counterparts. The impetus is on you to check and prepare, before you leave the U.S.

There are quite a few travel insurance companies and products. One type of travel insurance can be purchased for one trip, either at the point of flight sale or separately on the insurance website or in the insurance office. Trip insurance can cover a single episode or all trips over a time interval, such as a 6-month or one-year period. This insurance can cover only one travel claim service or several claim services, including trip cancelation, trip delay, emergency medical, evacuation, rental car, baggage delay and lost/stolen baggage. The most common type of trip cancelation insurance or trip cancelation clause will only cover unforeseen and named causes for cancelation, such as job loss, your illness or a death in the family. There are also a number of premium coverages that can be additionally purchased, such as coverage for pre-existing conditions or reimbursement of change fee and loyalty redeposit fee.

Some premier credit cards, with the purchase of all or some components of the trip, may cover some of these travel insurance features with variable terms and conditions. For example. American Express Platinum will cover trip cancelation or interruption up to $10,000 per covered trip and $20,000 per year, $500 twice a year for trip delays of at least 6 hours, and $75,000 if your rental car is stolen or in an accident and for lost or stolen luggage.

The COVID-19 pandemic led to many overseas travelers believing they were insured when they weren't. These returning overseas travelers were not reimbursed for medical and travel expenses. Travel insurance does not cover cancelations because of a pandemic. They will only cover costs if the unforeseen policy-named event such as illness, (even COVID-19 illness) occurred before the COVID-19 pandemic was known. For Allianz, "known" was January 22, 2020 and for Travel Guard it was March 11, 2020. So, a traveler would be reimbursed by Travel Guard but not Allianz for getting sick with COVID-19 and returning back to the U.S. on February 28, 2020.

Most standard travel insurance will not cover cancelations for government or community stay-at-home orders ("self-quarantine"), travel bans or other governmental restrictions on travel. Some travel insurers have offered to move coverage to the future rescheduled trip within, for example, 770 days. Travel insurers won't cover cancelation over fear. Fear over the possibility of getting ill would not trigger coverage. Only mandatory, enforced isolation would be covered for cancelation.

One option is to purchase a more costly "cancel for any reason" (CFAR) policy. There are not many of these CFAR policies available. If you do find one for your trip, it will usually cost you twice the standard travel insurance premium and offer less reimbursement per event. You would generally need to cancel, with the CFAR policy, 2-3 days before the flight and would likely be reimbursed 50-75% of your costs.

A couple remaining strategies are to self-insure or hedge purchases of flights. One option to self-insure for expensive flights is to purchase refundable tickets. These flights are pricier up front, but are fully reimbursable for a tenuously planned trip. Another strategy is to buy deep-discounted flights that won't be financially burdensome if canceled. Sometimes airlines will give a voucher, credit or change with a low fee, for a canceled flight. Travel insurance, credit card coverage benefits and travel spending strategies are all the moving parts in determining health security and holiday enjoyment during your next overseas trip.

References and Links

https://travel.state.gov/content/travel/en/international-travel.html

https://wwwnc.cdc.gov/travel/yellowbook/2020/health-care-abroad/travel-insurance-travel-health-insurance-and-medical-evacuation-insurance

https://www.allianztravelinsurance.com/travel/planning/unforeseen-event-coverage.htm

https://www.medicare.gov/coverage/travel

EX-PATRIOTS

Americans living abroad are often older and have existing or will develop medical problems while in another country. In addition, injuries can occur anywhere. It is estimated that a healthy 65-year-old retiree will spend over $250,000 on basic healthcare, from that point and through the remainder of their lives. Double that for a couple. This figure does not include prescription costs, which of course can be huge. It does not include the costs for dental or long-term care. Travel insurance will cover some emergency treatment and evacuation. Medicare will cover under limited circumstances. Medicare will not cover typical healthcare expenses overseas, as they would if living in the U.S.

There is a penalty for any 65-year-old not electing certain components of Medicare. This needs to be considered by those Americans living abroad, that turn 65 and eligible for Medicare. They would face a 10% premium penalty for every 12 months they are not enrolled in Part B outpatient services. There are penalties for late enrollments in other Medicare parts as well. Buying into Medicare, even while living outside the U.S., allows flexibility in the event of reunification for US-based healthcare.

There are a few other options that ex-patriots may need to consider when planning to live abroad. These include securing a separate International Health plan coverage through either a niche independent insurer or from a major American insurer. The latter are the same insurers that cover us domestically. Yet, these international plans will usually have limitations of coverage and higher cost sharing. Compared to their domestic counterparts, these international plans will cover less and cost more. Some overseas Americans will opt for lower-premium high-deductible catastrophic coverage.

Lowering living costs are one of the main reasons why ex-patriots ex-patriate. Managing healthcare and medical insurance costs are the highest priority motivations in these foreign relocations. Many ex-patriots will live out a period in their foreign country that allows buying into and receiving that country's national healthcare. Oftentimes, simply paying out of pocket, especially in countries with lower-cost healthcare services, is the most economical strategy either while waiting to be eligible for the country's healthcare coverage or as a permanent continuous healthcare purchasing strategy. Yet, lower healthcare costs need to be balanced with the quality of care in that country. Many Central and South American countries have low medical costs with good quality care.

An ex-patriot can often buy into the residing country's healthcare system. This can be done either as a visitor, temporary resident or becoming a full-fledged citizen and enjoying their social governmental healthcare system. Of course, each country will be different. Many counties deliver very good value for the taxes spent on health care. Some countries may have a long wait list for elective procedures and have inferior or indifferent care to those using the social healthcare program. Many countries have a formal or informal two-tiered health care system. Better healthcare services can be garnered by those privileged or with means (or even bribes). Those willing to spend more money and resources can enjoy better care, single-bed hospital rooms out of the hallway, and speedy services. Meshing into the country's national health care system may be easiest for those who hold dual citizenship.

The quality of health care in many popular ex-patriot destinations is actually quite good. Many are even considered better than the US. The popular ex-patriot European, Asian and Central and South American countries vary somewhat from year to year. Most popular destinations have a stable political system, pleasant climate and lower cost of living. The most popular European countries to live, in the last few years, are Spain, the Czech Republic and Portugal. France is considered to have the best healthcare system. Taiwan, Vietnam, Malaysia and Singapore are popular ex-patriot destinations, as is Bahrain. Mexico, Ecuador, Columbia, Panama and Costa Rica are havens for Americans. Italy, Greece and Brazil seem less favored today by U.S. ex-patriots. This is even though Italy is considered to have very good healthcare.

The most developed countries, such as in Northern Europe, Scandinavia and much of Asia have excellent healthcare systems. There is a greater cost of living to pay for these healthcare standards. Poorer counties tend to have less favorable national healthcare. But this is not always true of all Central and South American counties. Columbia is ranked above the U.S.

in health care. Brazil has a government universal healthcare system. Other countries with government-funded universal healthcare include Taiwan, Portugal, Spain, Greece, Italy and the UK. All the remaining countries have some other form of universal coverage, including employer-based with government safety nets.

An overseas country's universal healthcare does not always include the temporary or recent ex-patriot visitor, nor those who have acquired recent foreign citizenship. Costa Rica has modern state-of-the art facilities at about 1/3 of the U.S. costs. They provide universal coverage to all legal residents along with their citizens. Malaysia has very inexpensive health care delivered by Western-trained doctors, who speak English, in Joint Commission accredited facilities. Colombia does have public healthcare coverage but is so cheap that most ex-patriots simply pay out of pocket. Likewise, Mexico has good quality facilities with an abundance of American-trained Doctors. Mexico allows legal residents access to health care for about $300/year. Prescription drugs in Mexico are as low as 25% of what would be paid in the US.

"Free healthcare" is considered in the delivery, as no cost or a very minimal cost. The notion of overseas free healthcare being a free ride is not entirely true. Social healthcare is always funded in some way by the government, mostly through taxation, or by contributions from its industries and society. There may be cost sharing in these national coverages, co-pays and other fees. Bahrain, Canada,

France, Italy, Greece, Portugal, Singapore and Spain would be considered free under these definitions.

Legal residents or immigrants may have access to the universal coverage in their resident countries. But this is not widely true. Many countries do not let foreigners just walk into their universal healthcare programs. The rule is that nearly every country has open universal access for citizens and sometimes legal residents. It becomes more tenuous with lesser statuses, such as immigrants and refugees. Thailand is the only country that gives immigrants the same healthcare rights as citizens. Legal residents must buy into the universal health care of Germany and Greece.

It was realized during the recent period with large movement of people from Africa, the Middle East and other poorer parts of Europe and Eurasia, that most European countries do not readily open their healthcare systems to immigrants and refugees. Germany and Sweden give access for emergency services only. France and Portugal give full access to those even if illegal, after residing for 3 months. Legal residents may have access through the country's administrative processes.

Legal residents of other countries may also be able to purchase certain supplemental or catastrophic coverage in their newfound country. Often from U.S. Health insurers. Some maintain Medicare in order to hedge for a return back to the U.S. for certain healthcare needs. The decision for an ex-patriot to live in this or that country, and to become a resident or citizen, should put great consideration on the access to and quality of that country's healthcare.

References and Links

https://www.fidelity.com/viewpoints/personal-finance/plan-for-rising-health-care-costs

https://www.medicare.gov/coverage/travel

https://www.usnews.com/news/best-countries/slideshows/countries-with-the-most-well-developed-public-health-care-system

https://www.commonwealthfund.org/publications/newsletter-article/us-ranks-last-among-seven-countries-health-system-performance

https://www.numbeo.com/health-care/rankings_by_country.jsp

https://www.healthsystemtracker.org/chart-collection/health-spending-u-s-compare-countries/#item-spendingcomparison_gdp-per-capita-and-health-consumption-spending-per-capita-2019

MEDICAL TOURISM

Medical Tourism is specifically going to another country for the sole purpose of engaging in their healthcare services. Americans do this for a number of good reasons, including lower cost without sacrificing quality or originally immigrating from that country and seeking a procedure that is not available in the U.S. Other motivations may be speedier care or perceived better care, or even a more private setting for patient confidentially purposes. Americans go overseas for medical treatments ranging from butt-lifts to novel cancer therapy. The most common reasons for medical tourism are cosmetic surgery, dentistry and heart surgery.

Many of these countries market their welcoming clean modern facilities, English-speaking doctors and medical guidelines, as well as comfortable and delightful concierge services. These services can include luxury hotel stays and limousine pick-up and drop-off at the airports. Follow-up care needs to be arranged in the U.S. before leaving or upon return. Hopefully, a patient returns with accompanying medical records in English.

Medical tourists often travel to specific countries based on their reputation and expertise in certain procedures or treatments. Americans have been traveling for care at increasing rates, although the COVID pandemic did put a hold on this activity worldwide. Most Americans are traveling to Asian centers, which includes India, for overseas care. Most of the remaining American medical tourists go to

Central and South America. Canadians come to the U.S. at significant rates, avoiding long waits for their surgeries. Turkey is known for their inexpensive eye procedures. Mexico, as well as Poland and Hungary, are recognized for dentistry. Brazil and Thailand for cosmetic surgery. Thailand is known for its expertise in gender reassignment surgery. People travel overseas to India for orthopedic and cardiac procedures.

Health care outside the US is a buyer-beware consideration. Locations and services should be well researched. There are a number of organizations who can help in this research, including the non-profits Medical Tourism Association (MTA or Global Healthcare Organization) and Council on the Global Integration of Healthcare (CGIH). There is even medical tourism into the U.S. The Cleveland Clinic, Mayo Clinic and Johns Hopkins bring in well over a half million patients from outside the U.S., because of their specialization and expertise in orthopedics, cardiac care and oncology. So, it goes both ways.

The cost for medical tourism procedures and services can be astonishingly less than the cost in the U.S. For example, the World Health Organization (WHO) has shown that heart bypass surgery in the U.S. costs an average of $113,000 compared to $10,000 in India and $3250 in Mexico. Hip Replacement is $47,000 in the U.S., while costing around $11,000 in Thailand, Malaysia or Singapore and $6120 in Poland. First-class airfare from the U.S. to Europe can be easily found these days, for $2500 and to Asia for under $5000. Foreign luxury hotels are often under $100-200 a night. A one week stay in

Singapore or Poland, including luxury hotel and first-class flight for joint surgery would save about $30,000 to $38,000, respectively.

Beware of organ transplant tourism. Organ trafficking is the sale and purchase of human organs for transplantation. Some donors are those imprisoned in their country, who undergo forced organ harvest. Involuntary organ donation is estimated at 10% of all transplants. Kidneys are the most commonly harvested organs. This is because there is a supply-demand imbalance. There are typically over 100,000 Americans waiting for a kidney transplant, but there are under 20,00 kidney transplants each year. A significant portion of the remainder die while waiting.

A country's citizen traveling abroad to get a transplanted organ which was sold or coerced, is engaging in transplant tourism. One can argue that a sold organ can save another life. The problem is in the ethics and social imbalance. Human organs should not be considered a commodity. The World Health Organization, in their 1991 statement, indicated that organs should be preferentially removed from those deceased or voluntarily donated live from a genetically-related recipient. The Declaration of Istanbul on organ trafficking and transplant tourism creates unity consensus among countries against organ trafficking. The Istanbul Declaration distinguishes transplant "travel" from transplant "tourism." Travel relates to movement of donor, organ, recipient or professionals across borders to engage in professional medical transplantation. Travel becomes transplant tourism when it is a commercial process or undermines the ability to provide transplant services for its domestic population.

Other potential drawbacks of medical tourism are lower quality of care and lessening of continuity in follow-up care or observation. Complications from treatment abroad are not well known, usually recurring after returning to home countries and not revealed in introductory medical tourism marketing materials. There is also the loss of economic healthcare activity in the home countries, as some of the costliest services in a GDP are deflected outside.

Although seemingly counterintuitive, several small and large US healthcare insurers are covering and even promoting medical tourism, in order to lower some costs of what would otherwise be domestic care services. UnitedHealth Florida and three of the Blue Cross plans are allowing care to be delivered in India, Mexico and Thailand. They are even covering travel expenses. Medical tourism is increasing into and out of many countries, including the U.S. Our healthcare costs are well recognized as expensive with outcomes that do not align with these higher costs. In other words, U.S. healthcare is not a good value. Value is therefore being be found, increasingly, outside our borders.

References and Links
https://wwwnc.cdc.gov/travel/page/medical-tourism
https://www.medicaltourism.com/

https://journals.lww.com/transplantjournal/Full
Text/2013/06150/Organ_Trafficking_and_Transpla
nt_Tourism___The.2.aspx

CANADIAN & MEXICAN PHARMACEUTICALS

Prescription drug costs can be so great that some Americans will not fill prescriptions, will stretch out their prescriptions, share prescriptions or defer food and other essential expenses, in order to buy their prescriptions. Drug costs are higher in the U.S. than in every other country, and are increasing. For comparison, prescription spending per capita in our country is twice that of the United Kingdom. The causes for higher American drug costs include lack of price regulation and price transparency, relaxation of direct-to-consumer advertising stimulating prescription seeking, expansion of drug purchasing programs into many governmental programs and the business complexities of the pharmaceutical and health care supply chain. The federal government is currently pursuing price transparencies. All of these mentioned challenges are either absent or under better control in most other countries. The U.S. costs are higher despite using a greater proportional number of generics. The cost of Humira for Crohn's Disease and Rheumatoid arthritis in the U.S. is over $3000/dose. That is at least 3 times higher than in all of Europe and Canada.

U.S. Customs and Border Protection (CBP) and the Transportation Security Administration (TSA) agents operating the nation's airports have the regulatory authority to manage your medications into and out of the U.S. The CBP has certain restrictions on what can come back into this country, either as prescriptions crossing back over the borders or imported in by mail. It is technically illegal to bring prescriptions for personal use, purchased outside the U.S., back into this country. Instead, the FDA has guidance on how this can be finessed. The government is, essentially, turning a blind eye to the practice. No one has ever been prosecuted. It is a daily and widespread practice to bring back up to a 90-day supply of foreign prescription medicines back home.

One should have either the actual prescription coming back into the U.S., in its original instruction-labeled bottle, a valid written or printed prescription, or a doctor's note in English. Mail-order medications into the U.S. are mostly prohibited, since the FDA is not able to verify their safety and efficacy. The FDA, through its Personal Importation Policy, will allow a 90-day supply of medications otherwise illegal, to enter by mail only in order to treat a serious illness for which the U.S. does not have an effective treatment, as long as it would not cause an unreasonable health risk and is accompanied by a foreign doctor's letter in English.

Prescription drugs acquired in Canada and Mexico are much cheaper than the same drugs purchased in the U.S. American citizens in states neighboring Canada and Mexico have been crossing these borders, for this purpose, for many years. Canadian pharmacies will dispense if a U.S. border-crosser carries in a prescription or they will dispense after an on-site consultation and generated prescription. It has been reported that prescription drugs can be purchased in Mexico by simply walking into a Mexican pharmacy and purchasing. No questions asked. This prescription seeking outside the U.S. extends further than the individual citizen. Certain states and our federal government have considered their own trans-border purchases, in order to lower the cost to their constituents. The state of Utah employee health plan will fly their members to San Diego, under their Pharmacy Treatment Program, and transport them across the border into Tijuana for a 90-day supply of otherwise expensive prescriptions. The federal government, through some of its programs, has threatened bulk-drug purchasing from other counties.

In contrast, the FDA has myriad safeguards for prescription drugs purchased in the U.S. You can count on the safety and quality of an American pharmaceutical. That is not always true when purchasing drugs outside the country or through mail order. Narcotics and medications with high potential for abuse may never be brought back across the border. Novel treatments or devices, for example to cure cancer, cannot be brought back unless they are FDA-approved. Americans can only bring 50 doses of a controlled substance back, unless it was written by a U.S. Drug Enforcement Agency (DEA) registered physician. Only prescriptions that could otherwise be legally prescribed in the U.S. can be imported back from a Canadian or other foreign pharmacy. The FDA recently sent a warning letter to a Canadian company selling prescription drugs online to Americans. Another Canadian mail order pharmacy is deliberately misleading American consumers by implying the drugs are coming from Canada when, instead, these drugs are often coming from less-regulated Third World countries. Yet, another Canadian mail order pharmacy was found to have sold a counterfeit cancer drug.

Prescriptions drugs from across the border may seem quite a bargain. Care must be taken to confirm the quality and authenticity of any foreign prescription drug. Canada, New Zealand, Australia, and much of Western Europe have well-regulated pharmacies. Drugs elsewhere do not undergo the same regulation and oversight as those generated within the U.S. These foreign prescription drugs may even cause harm.

Prescription cost savings can still be found here in this country. American generics are often found to be cheaper than those purchased across the border. There are a few websites that scan U.S. medication prices. These website-based services are themselves bulk purchasers and use co-pay assistances that can lead to very low costs. A recent medication cost comparison with GoodRx found that Publix pharmacy has over 2-3x lower cost when compared to a health plan's pharmaceutic cost. These GoodRx drug costs beat Radiology Benefit Manager's (RBM) costs.

Certain medications such as Omeprazole for heartburn can be purchased off the shelf, from any drugstore or big box store. The prescription drug manufacturer will very often have programs for co-pay assistance. Co-pay assistance is intended to pay the portion of your cost-sharing for an expensive medication. The manufacturer of Humira can help lower the prescription cost from $3000 to a fraction. Beware though, one health plan and its Pharmacy Benefit Manager (PBM) is taking those co-pay assistance funds from the patient and pocketing them. This co-pay assistance is then not credited to the patient's deductible. One work-around to this is by the patient paying out-of-pocket for the entire pharmacy costs and then collecting the co-pay assistance directly from the drug manufacturer's program. U.S. prescription consumers, and their support services, are getting more and more creative to lower costs. This is happening while the U.S. pharmaceutical companies remain steadfast on their higher and increasing costs.

References and Links
https://www.webmd.com/healthy-aging/features/buying-drugs-across-border#1
https://www.fda.gov/industry/import-basics/personal-importation

HEALTHCARE OVERSIGHT & SCRUTINY

COVERAGE

The U.S. Center for Medicare and Medicaid Services (CMS) defines healthcare services coverage as the "legal entitlement to payment or reimbursement for your healthcare costs, generally under a contract with a health insurance company, a group health plan offered in connection with employment, or a government program like Medicare, Medicaid, or the Children's Health Insurance Program (CHIP)." Under the Affordable Care Act (ACA) all commercial insurers, including those self-funded, must supply the beneficiary a "Summary of Benefits and Coverage" (SBC) explaining their coverage in a standard fashion across compliant plans. An SBC must contain definitions of terms and examples with a description of the coverage, cost sharing, limitations and a phone number for further questions or to obtain a copy of the plan policy.

The ACA has certain requirements for health plan coverage, including pre-existing conditions, free-screening and maximums of spend without lifetime limits. The maximum cost sharing allowed under the ACA currently, also called Maximum Out-of-Pocket Spend (OOP) are $8150 for an individual and $16,300 for a family. This does not include the premium paid annually. The ACA health plan premium can be government subsidized, based on income. The ACA no longer allows lifetime or annual dollar spend limits. It was shocking when the pre-existing condition exclusion, with wait periods for coverage and lifetime limits, was instituted by health plans. This was challenging to the American consumer for a service vital to daily life, safety and productivity. In this way, health plans could collect several months premium without paying for services related to that pre-existing condition. As mentioned, the ACA did remove these clauses and then expanded health care insurance to those previously uninsured. These previously uninsured are primarily the working poor, who became insured with manageable or complete premium subsidies and, through many states, Medicaid expansions. It is noteworthy that preventative healthcare services through an ACA compliant plan, are delivered at no cost. These preventative services are categorized for each of the adult, woman and pediatric categories. For example, the adult free preventative services include lung cancer CT screening, depression or tobacco screening, and immunizations.

Coverage should be outlined in a way easy to understand and to engage in health care going forward, after review and reference to your health plan SBC. Yet, on occasion, you may complete a healthcare service, have your Provider bill for it, and then receive notification from your plan that the service is not covered. The health plan will send you an Explanation of Benefits (EOB), which is generated when your provider submits a claim for payment. The EOB will categorize what, if any, they will pay to that provider, what they will discount and your balance to be paid as cost sharing or non-coverage payment. You will be responsible for payment to be sent, not to the plan, but directly to the provider. This non-coverage may occur for several reasons, including lack of coverage on the policy, lack of medical necessity for the procedure, an excluded service or procedure on your policy or lack of getting prior authorization needed before that service or procedure occurred.

There are several straightforward and sometimes tricky reasons that require the patient to pay all or part of the bill. You may have a balance to pay designated on your EOB because you have some cost sharing, such as a co-pay or deductible that may be required after the bill has been discounted and paid to the provider. The reason for non-coverage could be that the service was deemed not medically necessary for your condition. For example, if you got an MRI of your back before your doctor tried some treatment for the pain. Another reason could be that the service was determined to be experimental or investigational (E&I). Proton-beam radiation, instead of using standard radiation techniques to shrink a tumor, is often considered E&I.

Surprisingly, non-coverage can occur due to a clerical error or inaccurate input of your medical condition. Clearing up these errors or misunderstandings is the easiest way to get non-coverage overturned. Another straightforward reason is that your coverage may have lapsed, or you are between insurance plans and your service did not occur during the insured period. The coverage could have been out-of-network or by an out-of-network provider. You may have to cost-share more or pay the entire amount.

This can happen with surprise-billing, when you go into an in-network hospital facility for an outpatient colonoscopy and receive a bill for the full amount for the biopsy pathology reading. This happens because, even though the facility and provider doing the colonoscopy are in-network, the pathologist is not. Unfortunately, you have no way of knowing this up front. Finally, your treatment may have required a prior authorization before getting the service. Prior authorization means that your provider needs to submit enough information to satisfy medical necessity and coverage prior to certain services, such as expensive medications or high-technology imaging. If you don't agree with a denied service, you have rights to both an internal and external appeal. Internal is within the plan and external is by an outside independent-review entity.

References and Links
https://www.healthcare.gov/health-care-law-protections/summary-of-benefits-and-coverage/
https://www.medicare.gov/forms-help-resources/mail-you-get-about-medicare/explanation-of-benefits-eob

COST-SHARING (CO-PAYS, DEDUCTIBLES, CO-INSURANCE, OUT-OF-POCKET MAXIMUMS)

Cost sharing is the amount of money the health plan beneficiary pays out-of-pocket for their health care. This occurs with most both employer and government health plans. There are a couple of reasons for cost sharing. Bearing some personal cost for health care creates an obvious personal pain point and will therefore theoretically limit you to seek only the most appropriate care. You would hold off on getting less vital and less urgent healthcare.

Probably, the major reason for cost sharing is that your employer gets to pass part of the burden of financing your healthcare, onto you. Cost sharing includes deductibles, coinsurance, and copayments. Cost sharing does not include premiums, balance billing amounts for non-network providers, or the cost of non-covered services. Cost sharing does though, include the health insurance premium paid for Medicaid and Children's Health Insurance Plan (CHIP).

The monthly premium is either paid directly by the individual policy holder to the health plan or shared with the employer, with the member's portion taken out of the employment paycheck. Health plans with lower monthly premiums will almost always have higher deductibles. Plans with higher monthly premiums will have lower deductibles. You can see this with the ACA plans from Bronze, Silver to Gold.

Medicare Part B can be deducted from the Social Security benefit. There are very few plans today that give the employee a full ride; the so-called Cadillac plan. In other words, no cost-sharing for services. The employment health insurance benefit is considered a salary-equivalent portion of the employment income package. So, if you didn't get health insurance, your salary should be higher. Cost sharing has increased as health insurance prices have increased. Those with health insurance through the ACA may have premium cost reduction based on income. The ACA also offers cost-sharing reduction for those that qualify on their Silver plan or for Native American or Alaskan Natives.

Your insurer has negotiated with certain providers at in-network rates. While those providers that do not join the plan are considered out-of-network. Your cost sharing will be different toward each of these sets of services. Your health plan may have a 20% coinsurance for an in-network provider but a 50% coinsurance for an out-of-network provider. Through this, your health plan prefers you to use the in-network providers.

Copayment is a fixed amount that a subscriber pays for a healthcare service. It is collected directly from you out-of-pocket at the time of or soon after the service. This amount, paid for a specific medical service, is set by your insurer and can vary by each plan offered by that insurer and other insurers. This copay for a service may be required even after you pay and fulfill your deductible amount, that is until you reach your annual total out-of-pocket amount. Yet, most co-payments do not count towards the deductible. A co-payment example would be an ER visit for stomach pain. This service requires you to pay the hospital or clinic a set amount of $50 for that visit. The insurer pays the rest.

Your coinsurance requirement kicks in after you have paid your annual deductible. It is a percentage of the amount that the insurer allows to be charged for that service. So, let's say you have engaged in services through the year paying your portion throughout. That portion you have paid now meets your $5000 deductible. You are not quite done with cost sharing. Coinsurance for your next trip to the ER with a headache, this time, would require you to pay, for example, 30% of the cost for that ER visit. Your insurer would pay the other 70%. That would be a 30% coinsurance payment instead of the co-pay that you would have previously paid. Co-payments are on the front end of health insurance services. While, coinsurance comes on the back end, after meeting the deductible.

The deductible is the amount you pay for healthcare services out-of-pocket before your health insurance begins to start paying full costs. Deductibles only apply to money you spend on covered services that are billed to the insurance plan. An example could be seeing an Orthopedist for ankle pain. That Provider bills and is paid $250 by your health plan. You then pay the remaining $50 of the total $250 bill. That $50 then is counted towards your annual deductible amount. Several more visits and services through the year, would include further similar patient payments, up to the deductible amount for individual or family.

Once you meet the family deductible all members no longer need to meet the individual deductible. The health plan starts paying all for anyone and everyone, except for any required copays or co-insurance. This also works at the individual level. The health plan starts paying all for one member if that member is the first to meet their deductible This occurs for that member even if the family deductible has not yet been met.

Cold medicines bought over-the-counter, off the shelf at a drug store would not count toward your deductible since you paid cash and there was no claim for payment sent to your insurer. It is not a health plan covered product. Copays are not included toward the deductible. There may be some services, like preventative care, which do not count towards your deductible for that plan. Free services do not count toward your deductible. For example, an office visit and swab test for COVID-19 is a required free service to you. Your health plan still pays the provider. But no cost of that free service is applied toward your deductible.

Cost sharing is more clearly illustrated with a Health Savings Account. Let's say that trip to the ER cost $1500 and your deductible is $1500. You would pay all of that $1500 out-of-pocket or from your Health Savings Account. The provider doesn't care how they are paid. After this, you would not need to pay toward any deductible for the rest of that year.

Out-of-pocket (OOP) maximum is the absolute maximum you pay out of your own pocket for any cost sharing during that plan year. This always occurs after your deductible has been met. Any further coinsurance payments would contribute toward the OOP maximum. You are no longer required to make any further out-of-pocket payments, including copays, deductible or coinsurance, once you have met the OOP maximum amount.

The States' Medicaid plans may impose limited or higher premiums for certain groups of members. Institutionalized individuals and most children are excluded from Medicaid cost-sharing requirements. The states may establish different co-payments for generic versus brand-name drugs and higher copays for non-preferred drugs for those with higher income levels. Emergency services are exempted from all out-of-pocket charges in Medicaid. States can impose higher co-payments for ER visits for non-emergency services. Medicare Part A (hospital services) is generally premium-free. Otherwise Medicare does require variable cost sharing and premium payment for other parts and services. Likewise, Medicare Advantage plans share the same features as commercial cost-sharing plans.

References and Links

https://www.healthcare.gov/

https://www.medicaid.gov/medicaid/cost-sharing/index.html

https://www.medicare.gov/your-medicare-costs/medicare-costs-at-a-glance

NETWORK

The health plan sets rates for your provider's goods and services, for them to bill for your services. The provider or facility becomes "in-network" if they accept the insurer's set rates. These in-network providers or facilities are then contractually eligible to provide services to you for that health plan. Eligibility may be due to the provider credentialing or the need for that healthcare service in the health plan's network. Credentialing of these providers by the health plan, also call Provider Enrollments, is the review of education, training, and professional experience. Health insurance companies are required to publish web-based lists of in-network providers for their plans, so that this information is accessible to the subscribers. A provider or facility is considered "out-of-network" if they are still undergoing credentialing, did not apply to that health plan or did not agree to the insurer's rates.

Depending on your insurance plan, you may have no coverage for out-of-network care, or you may have to pay higher co-insurance costs and meet a higher out-of-network deductible, if you see a provider or get services at a facility that does not participate with your insurer. In other words, out-of-network. You may also end up paying the difference between what the doctor charges for a specific procedure and what your health insurer is willing to pay for that care. It not just the increased cost sharing associated with out-of-network health care. This out-of-network provider may not accept the rate paid to them by the insurer and bill you for the balance or the entire amount. You would then have to send a claim yourself, to your insurer to get back the out-of-network rate reimbursement. In this example, since your provider totally refused payment from the insurer, any balance in either situation would be your responsibility.

There are few ways that you may be able to get the in-network rate or at least a discount on the out-of-network rate, after seeing an out-of-network provider. The first is called a "network gap exception" and involves reaching out to your health plan, requesting an in-network payment, for an out-of-network provider, because of extenuating circumstances. These circumstances include your inability to get the get the care you need because your insurer's narrow network doesn't include any physician who offers the essential medical service you need. The insurers will often allow this if you are requesting a covered service that is medically necessary but not offered by an in-network provider in your region. If the insurer does this, then you will not have to pay the larger difference for out-of-network services. Other reasons that you may get an exception from out-of-network fees, are emergency care that did not allow seeking in-network care or you were not aware that the urgent or emergent facility or provider was out-of-network when the injury or symptoms arose. Finally, another reason to request an exemption is that your provider changed status from in to out-of-network during a course of treatment.

Some doctors or facilities may be willing to discount the overall services they provided if you are willing instead, to pay them out-of-pocket upfront, instead of going through insurance. In fact, that discount could be less than your cost sharing and balance billing amount. That out-of-pocket payment may not be applied to your deductible and maximum out-of-pocket. That is, unless you billed and collected from the insurer directly.

Another option on the back end is to negotiate down a bill payment required. Some providers and facilities may look sympathetically at a large bill and discount 20%, or even up to 50% if you are under difficult financial straits. You can do this yourself or through a paid financial patient advocacy service. The best strategy to avoid or mitigate the hassle and higher out-of-pocket costs is to choose a plan that includes the providers and facilities that you plan to use. This is done during the next open-enrollment period or if you have an event, such as loss of employment health insurance, and are transitioning to another health plan.

References and Links
https://www.patientadvocate.org/explore-our-resources/understanding-health-insurance/out-of-network-costs-and-how-to-handle-them-2/

BILLING

Billing for healthcare services is usually done by the provider or facility where services are rendered. This is a claim sent to your insurer. The provider requires you to sign a release that allows them to bill your healthcare insurer for these services in your place. Health insurance claims filed with carriers by providers on behalf of policyholders are almost entirely handled electronically. The insured member may, on occasion, have to file a claim directly to the insurer if the provider is out-of-network or does not accept your insurance. That way you can at least get personally reimbursed the out-of-network amount.

The provider creates a "superbill" with information about the provider, you and the service. This superbill is submitted as a claim by either themselves or through a clearinghouse. This claim sent electronically is required to include an ICD code (International Classification of Disease) for the diagnosis and a CPT code (Current Procedural Terminology) for the level of service or procedure. CMS (Center for Medicare and Medical Services) and a few insurers use HCPCS codes (Healthcare Common Procedural Coding System) instead of CPT codes. HCPCS codes describe services not found in the CPT, including non-physician services, such as ambulance, durable medical equipment, and prescription drug use.

The medical billing and coding cycle can take from a few days to several months. At times, a high fee for services claimed will be reviewed by the insurer, for medical necessity coverage. A denied claim can be rectified and appealed. The in-network provider would then get paid for the in-network agreed upon fee for that service. You would then need to pay that provider any copay or deducible not covered in the settlement by the insurer of that claim. Increasing cost sharing, especially the huge contributions required by the insured into an HSA, have led to half of all patients unable or unwilling to pay all of their balance to providers or facilities. An additional and unpleasant back-end request for payment can also be by an out-of-network provider or facility, called "surprise" or "balance" billing. As with any other businesses, delinquent medical debts can be managed by or sold to collection agencies.

References and Links
https://www.ama-assn.org/practice-management/claims-processing

SURPRISE & BALANCE BILLING

Twenty to 50% of all ER visits lead to a medical bill or bills for services that were believed to be lower cost in-network care, but are billed to the patient at a higher or full cost rate for these services. Because all or some components of that care were not in-network. This can occur with any other healthcare service, such and endoscopy or biopsy. This situation is referred to as 'surprise" medical billing and is on the increase. It can also be called "balance billing," since the insurer is leaving to you the responsibility of the unpaid balance, not paid to them by the insurer, for their out-of-network charge. You are then on the hook to pay the provider, hospital or clinic, this balance unpaid by the health plan.

Surprise or balance billing occurs because prospective in-network providers negotiate and accept in-network rates for healthcare services. All other provider's services are then "out-of-network." The out-of-network providers and their services are not required to set a price. Out-of-network and direct patient billing is always at a much higher rate.

The surprise bill payment request will be the patient's responsibility even if the hospital is in the insurer's network. This is exactly when the insured gets blindsided. A specific doctor may be delivering out-of-network services from an in-network hospital. A typical example of surprise billing can occur during an elective screening colonoscopy. The patient enters the in-network facility and receives the colonoscopy by an in-network gastroenterologist. Sedation is given to you also by an in-network anesthesiologist. Your recovery is conducted by in-network hospital employed nurses. Yet, the polyp biopsy taken during that colonoscopy results in a sizeable complete bill sent to you the patient because the pathologist's biopsy evaluation services are not in-network. Even in an in-network facility.

Doctors are increasingly becoming hospital employees. Yet, there are still quite a few doctors in independent or group practices that also serve patients within the hospital or clinic. It is the higher-charging specialist that tends to be out-of-network, and unfortunately more often become the surprise billers. These include anesthesiologists which surprise bill an average of 5.5x higher than Medicare charges. Emergency Medicine, Pathology and Radiology specialists also send a high amount of surprise bills, with charges 4x higher than Medicare. This is contrasted with the almost non-existent surprise bills sent by Primary Care physicians.

The reason why these specialists are out-of-network is dissatisfaction with in-network rates. This conflict between certain specialists and insurers leaves you stuck with the bill over their disputes. Yet, there are some strategies in dealing with surprise bills. The vast majority of surprise bills are very inflated. Surprise bills can be in excess of what any insurer or Medicare would pay; most are 2-3x times higher. The provider sets their rates deliberately high in order to capture the highest insurance payer. That leaves those with surprise bills with the highest bill amount from that provider. The insurer would never pay this amount. The patient should not pay this amount either.

These surprise bills can be frequently negotiated lower by either the patient or through a paid private service. Some states will allow you to collect payment from the insurer for the out-of-network charge. You can use the out-of-network amount to negotiate down the charge from the surprise biller, to satisfy payment obligation. Thankfully, some hospitals are requiring all providers on staff to accept in-network payments whether they are in or out of network.

Lawmakers are discussing protections, as this practice increases and more patients complain or refuse to pay surprise bills. Insurers and hospitals/providers, both sides on this matter, have significant financial resources to hire lobbyists and launch publicity campaigns to position themselves favorably, concerning any prospective legislation. The providers have appeared more sympathetic to the public, since they are the doing the work, providing the care. The insurers are less sympathetic.

One suggestion is to lower out-of-network rates. Out-of-network rates can be examined in two ways. One is through arbitrations between insurers and providers, to set a payment for each service. This is the doctor's preferred approach. The other way to set out-of-network rates and is preferred by the payers. This solution could be to benchmark the price by using median in-network rate for the out-of-network service. This benchmark option is also preferred by large employers and labor unions, who are the payers of the group benefits. Surprise billing has been increasing steadily over the last several years. The increasing public outrage associated with this increase in surprise billing is getting the attention of these constituency's lawmakers.

Lastly, surprise or balance billing needs to be distinguished from "post-claim underwriting." Post-claim underwriting is a process of reviewing the medical necessity of a service after that claim has been submitted to that health plan. This can occur with both in or out-of-network services. The insurer delays paying this claim to the provider, until they are satisfied that the service is covered or not excluded from coverage. This was seen quite often when pre-existing conditions were excluded from some coverages. Before the ACA. The post-claim underwriting review can lead to payment of the claim at the in or out-of-network rate if coverage and/or medical necessity is determined. There will be no payment at all, if deemed not coverage or not medically necessary.

References and Links
https://www.kff.org/private-insurance/fact-sheet/surprise-medical-bills-new-protections-for-consumers-take-effect-in-2022/

HEALTH INSURANCE PORTABILITY AND ACCOUNTABILITY ACT (HIPAA)

The Healthcare Insurance Portability and Accountability Act (HIPAA), first created in 1996, has undergone several modifications and amendments in order to adapt to the evolving electronic world today. The original Act was signed by President Clinton into law in order to have the Secretary of Health and Human Services (HHS) create regulations for healthcare privacy and security standards, and deeming responsibility of protecting the privacy by covered entities, health plans, and healthcare clearinghouses. "Portability" means that the patient's medical record information should move easily from health plan to health plan, and provider to provider. The "accountability" aspect ensures that this patient's medical record passes and is accessed with privacy and confidentiality. The medical records producers, transporters and custodians, as Covered Entities and their Business Associates must comply, and are on the hook, for this portability and accountability.

The most important addition was the Omnibus Rule of 2013, which included employees, volunteers, trainees, and other persons who perform work for a Covered Entity or Business Associate, as under the direct management of the Covered Entity or Business Associate, also must adhere to the HIPAA protected information and identifiers of confidentiality. It should be noted that persons or organizations, such as social media participants (e.g., Facebook, etc.) and those engaging in community public health behaviors (e.g., airlines requiring masks during COVID-19) are neither HIPAA Covered Entities nor their Business Associates. So, these social media and public health individual and business are not required to maintain other's health and medical privacy. They are not restricted from asking an individual question about their health. Only entities described within this act must comply with its privacy and security standards and processes.

HIPAA improved with time. The HIPAA Privacy Rule became effective in 2003, which improved privacy standards and restricted disclosure of Protected Health Information (PHI) and personal identifiers, to only those unauthorized. The Privacy Rule gave patients improved access to their health information. The Security Rule became effective two years later in 2005, further protecting this individual health information shared by those authorized. The next year saw the 2006 HIPAA Breach Enforcement Rule, giving the Office for Civil Rights (OCR) the authority to enforce the HIPAA Rules through financial penalties against non-compliant entities. The Health Information Technology for Economic and Clinical Health Act ("HITECH" Act) of 2009, as part of the American Recovery and Reinvestment Act (ARRA), gave providers incentives to switch from paper to electronic health records (EHR), also called electronic medical records (EMR). That same year saw the enforcement of HIPAA strengthening, with the Breach Notification Rule, requiring Covered Entities to report data breaches to OCR, and then to the breached individuals. That year also led to the Enforcement Rule for tiered financial penalties, with fines increased to $1.5 million per violation. The final Omnibus Rule became effective in 2013, adding direct liability for business associates, indefinite security of data storage, and taking into account changing work practices with the widening use of mobile devices.

The early years saw little if any enforcement. More recently that has changed, with the use of audits, greater financial penalties, sanctions, potential loss of licensure and even criminal convictions. HIPAA has been a major step in protecting your medical data and making those accountable for that protection, even if its reach and power is often misunderstood and over asserted by the public at large.

References and Links
https://www.hhs.gov/hipaa/index.html
https://www.healthit.gov/topic/privacy-security-and-hipaa/hipaa-basics
https://www.hipaajournal.com/hipaa-history/

PRIOR AUTHORIZATION

The health plan insurer pays for services for you, called a subscriber, member or beneficiary covered under that plan. Healthcare services covered must be deemed medically necessary for a commercial plan, or "reasonable and necessary" for Medicare. Its essentially the same. Both commercial and governmental insurers undergo some types of internal review to determine medical necessity coverages. In other words, there must be an appropriate and covered clinical reason for that healthcare service.

Appropriateness or medical necessity for that healthcare service can be satisfied through physician examination, likely diagnosis, labs study results or other radiology results. Medical necessity coverage is needed for every healthcare service, treatment plan, durable medical equipment and prescription drug. A claim is a request for payment for goods or services delivered to a health plan beneficiary, by a provider to the health plan. The vast majority of claims for low cost covered healthcare services quickly pass through and are paid, without verifying medical necessity. Yet, nearly all of the higher cost services are scrutinized for medical necessity.

These higher cost services will usually undergo "prior authorization," also called pre-authorization, prior approval or pre-certification. Prior authorization is a utilization management strategy for reviewing medical necessity appropriateness, using a set of guidelines or criteria, with the theory that this process improves safety and lowers costs. Like all intermediaries in healthcare, prior authorization comes at a cost. A cost to both the member and provider. Since, prior authorization has demonstrated improvement in patient safety and cost savings for members.

Prior authorization requires your provider to get approval from either the health plan or the health plan's benefit manager, before prescribing a high-cost medication or service or procedure. These include CT scans, MRIs, PET scans, sleep studies, and now endoscopies. The health plan will often do the prior authorization in-house. They increasingly will contract this out to a vendor or delegate, usually a benefit manager. These benefit manager's revenues have increased over time, to become attractive acquisition targets. Cigna bought the Pharmacy Benefit Manager (PBM) Express Scripts, one year after Express Scripts bought the Radiology Benefit Manager (RBM) eviCore. Magellan owns the RBM, National Imaging Associates. Another RBM, called AIM, is owned by Anthem.

Your health plan will not pay the provider's claim for a service rendered without prior authorization approval, if required for that healthcare good or service. The health plan member who received that unapproved completed service will then be billed by that provider, the full amount for that service. That is unless you and the provider are able to backtrack with submission of information back to the health plan or delegate, to get a retroactive approval for that completed service. A retroactive approval may or may not be available, based on time passed since service completed, state laws and health plan policies.

The retrospective review is therefore a process of determining coverage, and payment for the claim, after services are rendered. This can occur because the procedure was thought not to require prior authorization. Or because the service occurred too quickly after being ordered, without available time to get prior authorization. This can occur, for example, after a member undergoes an appropriate mammogram that finds a suspicious spot. The Radiologist may suggest an immediate adjunctive breast ultrasound. The ultrasound request will not have gone through standard prior authorization. Otherwise, this request would require a day or two for normal prior authorization processing. This ultrasound payment request by the radiologist may then be rejected. Yet, in this case the ultrasound could be approved and paid through a retrospective process, assuming the need is medical necessary.

The need for prior authorization can vary from health plan to health plan, or lines of business within a health plan. Prior authorization can also be currently required by a health plan's line of business, when it was not required one month before. So, it is tricky to know from day-to-day which health plans or lines of their business requires prior authorization review. This needs to be continuously monitored by the provider's office and their healthcare ordering staff. This along with the entire prior authorization processing, which can often include provider peer-to-peer outreaches to the plan or benefit manager, creates what many providers consider an administrative burden and delays or interrupts care.

References and Links

https://www.ama-assn.org/amaone/prior-authorization?gclid=EAIaIQobChMIoLWyoNnB7wIV aUpyCh3w0Q8nEAAYAiAAEgIKs_D_BwE

https://www.commonwealthfund.org/publicatio ns/explainer/2019/apr/pharmacy-benefit-managers-and-their-role-drug-spending

https://www.jacr.org/article/S1546-1440(10)00684-8/pdf

QUALITY IMPROVEMENT ORGANIZATIONS (QIO)

The Center for Medicare and Medicaid Services Quality Improvement Organization (QIO) Program, is intended to improve health quality for Medicare beneficiaries, while doing this at a lower cost. This program is therefore intended to drive value for Medicare beneficiaries. One of a number of QIOs across the nation are designated for each state. These QIOs, which are independent and mostly non-profit private organizations, are staffed by health care professionals and quality improvement experts working to improve the quality and efficiency of health care across all care settings, especially hospital care.

There are two types of QIOs, described as Quality Innovation Network-QIOs (QIN-QIOs) and Beneficiary and Family Centered Care-QIOs (BFCC-QIOs). The 14 QIN-QIOs improve patient safety, reduce harm by engaging community providers, their patients and families by reducing certain health conditions in priority populations and preventing hospital readmissions. These QIO oversight duties for Medicare include pay for performance, disease management and accountability measures. The two

BFCC-QIOs help Medicare beneficiaries exercise their right to high-quality health care with their complaints, reviews, appeals and other cases in order to assert their right to high-quality health care. They address Medicare related complaints, such as beneficiary complaints, provider appeals and violations of the Emergency Medical Treatment and Labor Act (EMTALA).

References and Links
https://www.cms.gov/Medicare/Quality-Initiatives-Patient-Assessment-Instruments/QualityImprovementOrgs
https://www.qioprogram.org/locate-your-qio

BENEFIT MANAGEMENT

PHARMACY BENEFIT MANAGEMENT

A pharmacy benefit manager (PBM) is a private company that administers the drug benefit program for private health insurers, Medicare Part D drug plans and large employers. They tier drugs into certain payment categories and create processes for prescription access and delivery, such as through mail order. The RBM buys medications in large volumes from the drug companies, through discounts and negotiation of rebates back to the RBM. The RBMs maintain formularies that direct higher cost medications into specialty pharmacy services and leave some medications completely off the formularies. The RBM also ensures member compliance to medications and processes pharmacy claims.

There is increasing scrutiny about the RBM role in rising prescription drug costs and drug spending. Various reforms, at both the federal and state levels, have been suggested in order to bring RBMs back into the mission of creating better prescription drug value for the health plan members. These reforms include greater transparency of the rebates RBMs receive from drug makers and transferring those rebates into savings for health plan members, rather than RBMs pocketing the windfalls themselves. The other financial maneuvering that enhances RBM's revenues, is "spread pricing." Spread pricing occurs when the RBM keeps the difference between what the health plan pays for prescription drugs and what the RBM pays for those pharmacy services. RBMs do not pass the full payments received for these services, to the pharmacies. RBMs are one of a number of intermediary services, usually benefit managers, that creates another layer of cost, without clearly identified benefits to the health plan subscriber.

References and Links

https://www.commonwealthfund.org/publications/explainer/2019/apr/pharmacy-benefit-managers-and-their-role-drug-spending

https://www.pcmanet.org/the-value-of-pbms/

RADIOLOGY BENEFIT
MANAGEMENT

Radiology Benefit Managers (RBMs) are akin to PBMs, but instead of drugs, the RBM reviews and manages advance radiology service requests. RBMs are widely used by private health insurers, including their government administered Medicare Advantage plans. They also directly contract with state's Medicaid programs. The RBM is in place to manage what is believed to be over-utilization of imaging services, through their prior authorization. The RBMs have moved beyond medical imaging and into laboratory services, medical devices, chemotherapy and radiation therapy services, endoscopy and sleep apnea testing.

RBMs and PBMs intermediaries now reach into every aspect of our healthcare. Healthcare services are reviewed by the RBM, and either approved or denied. This is based on their set of medical necessity criteria. Criteria that often, but not always aligns with the health plan coverage policies. After approval, the member can then get that service. The member with the denied request will not be able to get that service without further review and determination. It is critical to understand that even though the RBM is the health plan delegate in these reviews, an RBM approved service request does not guarantee health plan payment. The denied service, if performed or performed without or before going through the authorization process, will be billed by the provider or facility directly to the health plan member. This leaves the entire cost of service the responsibility of the member. Therefore, it is in the member's best interest to be aware of the prior authorization policies of their health plan.

RBMs will charge health plans either on a per case request basis or the RBM will assume the full risk of that health plan coverage determination. One could anticipate the RBMs, if covering the risk, would be incentivized toward more denials. RBMs are criticized as "denial mills." Like PBMs, they do create more administrative work and costs for the provider. These increased healthcare costs ultimately lead to incremental increases in annual premiums for the health plan member.

Despite this impact on providers, the RBMs reach has increased, more and more, into US healthcare. Nearly every major RBM has been acquired by a large healthcare corporation. Unfortunately, the addition of this intermediary has not been shown, beyond anecdotal vignettes, to improve the health and safety of healthcare members. Nor is there evidence that costs have decreased because of RBM interventions.

References and Links

https://www.ama-assn.org/amaone/prior-authorization?gclid=EAIaIQobChMIoLWyoNnB7wIV aUpyCh3w0Q8nEAAYAiAAEgIKs_D_BwE

https://www.jacr.org/article/S1546-1440(10)00684-8/pdf

APPEAL

Any denial of coverage can get another look at approval of coverage for that healthcare good or service. This additional review of medical necessity coverage and/or payment, can happen even more than once. If you believe the service should be covered, either based on the plan's coverage documents or appropriate medical necessity, then the provider and/or the health plan member can appeal to the health plan or its benefit manager delegate.

It is particularly helpful if you have your provider supports and even orchestrates the appeal. It is less successful if the service was patient-driven with marginal appropriateness or benefit. This is important because the health plan will often reach out to the provider in this redetermination or appeal process. Many providers have had experience in dealing with health plans and their coverages for their specific and frequently ordered specialty services. They know which plans will cover or overturn an appeal for that service.

Appeals are part of any commercial or governmental health plan. They will include at least one internal appeal and one external appeal review. An internal review is done by an agent, usually a Medical Director employee, of that health plan or benefit manger. Often, with a different doctor from your denial, and usually a specialist. The external appeal review will be done by an outside party to the plan, for which the state or federal government has delegated to this task. Medicare uses a contractor called Maximus. State Medicaid appeals may be deferred to their Administrative Law Judge.

This appeal after the initial health plan denial, can have one of several different names. These include "re-determination," "additional review," "reconsideration," "reopen," "restart" or appeal, all at various levels. Most re-determinations or appeals require your provider to submit contemporaneous or new supporting documentation. The provider may engage in a "peer-to-peer" (P2P) discussion with the health plan or benefit manager's doctor. Oftentimes the P2P will lead to a meeting-of-minds and approval of the service. Most appeals tend to be overturned and approved. Some will stay denied.

There are several arguments to overturn a denial:

Health plan policies do cover
Benefit manager guidelines or criteria do cover
Request is reasonable (usually during P2P)
Vague health plan or benefit manager criteria
Community or politically supported emerging technology
Not Experimental and Investigational
VIP patient or family
Social media or state complaint noise

The health plan or benefit manager may have failed to identify that coverage or criteria may have actually been met. The electronic medical record is complicated and crowded. Mistake do occur. Interestingly, many times these RBM-adopted guidelines do not align with the health plan coverage for that service. This sort of mismatch can allow you to pick and choose between the health plan policy or benefit management guidelines to get your service approved. Although, benefit-management approval of any service is not a guarantee of payment. Simply because of this mismatch mentioned. But this should really never happen as too unfair to the beneficiary. Your state insurance commission handles complaints about your health plan or benefit manager. This and negative social media commentary get immediate attention from the health plan and benefit manager.

A service denial is very unlikely to be overturned if it is firmly considered "Experimental and Investigation" (EI), by either the health plan or benefit manager. EI means that there is no compelling scientific or systematic clinical evidence that this service is beneficial and without undue harm or risk. Most covered services have settled research and practice. Many EI procedures and services are new or dubious technologies. Sometimes new procedures or services are deemed EI because of high costs or a spike of requests.

One of the most common routes to overturn, if not the most common, is during the P2P conversation. There is a collegiality between doctors, whether within or across systems. Doctors spend all day discussing cases and referring patients to each other. The P2P reviewing doctor has significant leeway in approval. Some will often use a reasonableness of care standard. Others will approve as long as the treatment is not obviously harmful. A few may remain hardliners and uphold the denial.

Finally, the second or last level appeal will be through an independent review organization (IRO) always utilizing a same-specialty doctor. In other words, a doctor that specializes in medicine related to your continued denied request for goods or services. The external review process of health plan decisions, for all states, needs to meet the federal consumer protection standards. These provisions require that the health plan send written notice to the beneficiary who then has 40 days to reply. The IRO will then have 45 days, if not otherwise expedited, to send a binding response. The state may have an IRO process that exceeds the federal standards. The health plan must then accept this IRO decision.

References and Links
https://www.healthcare.gov/appeal-insurance-company-decision/appeals/
https://www.hhs.gov/healthcare/about-the-aca/cancellations-and-appeals/appealing-health-plan-decisions/index.html
https://www.medicare.gov/claims-appeals/how-do-i-file-an-appeal

EDUCATION & CREDENTIALING

PRE-MEDICAL BACCALAUREATE

Entry into medical school requires any undergraduate baccalaureate degree that satisfies a set of specific coursework, usually called "pre-medical" required courses. This specific coursework is required for the pre-medical ("pre-med") student to apply to each selected medical school. Yet, the degree major does not have to be in biology or other related sciences. A pre-med is welcome to major in, for example, mathematics, English, philosophy or psychology. Medical schools are looking for well-rounded individuals. Biochemistry, psychology and sociology courses are additionally important, because this knowledge base has been included into the Medical College Admission Test® (MCAT®), since 2015. There are no real barriers to medical school for qualified applicants. There is no age restriction to medical school matriculation. Quite a few applicants are in their 40s, 50s and even 60s.

The student will have to complete this pre-med courses, also called pre-requisites. Most medical schools require pre-requisites of one year of biology, general chemistry, organic chemistry and physics, all with their associated academic laboratories. Biochemistry and English are frequently pre-requisites for medical school applications.

Medical school admission is competitive. A grade point average (GPA) below 3.0 would generally not be considered for selection. A GPA between 3.6-4.0 will often ensure admission to a U.S. medical school. Medical schools will review your overall GPA and also consider a subset of biology, chemistry, physics, and math (BCPM) course grades.

All medical schools require the MCAT, which is administered several times each year. The MCAT should be completed no later than the summer following the junior year, so that medical school application will be considered during the fall of the student's senior year. The average MCAT score of successful applicants is 510 of a total possible 528. Scores of 518 or more are exceptional; those below 508 are not competitive for entry into allopathic medical schools. The MCAT can be repeated up to three times in one year, four times over a two-year period and retaken up to seven times in a lifetime. Medical schools will be aware of the multiple exam scores and use this as an average or acknowledge only the highest score, during their evaluations.

Clinical activities, research, teaching, extra-curricular and employment experiences can enhance a medical school application. All this information is collected and distributed through the American Association of Medical Colleges platform clearinghouse. Thereafter the application will be considered and either denied or lead to further steps taken. These further steps may include a secondary application to be submitted to that specific medical school or an in-person (or video) interview. Medical school acceptance rates have been decreasing over the last 20 years, to well under 10%. Medical school, residency and medical practice, which follows successful matriculation, are no less grueling. Nevertheless, a career in medicine and healthcare will have great rewards and satisfaction, in the improving of health and well-being of the population.

References and Links
https://students-residents.aamc.org/applying-medical-school/applying-medical-school-process/medical-school-admission-requirements/
https://www.aafp.org/students-residents/medical-students/considering-medical-school/getting-into-medical-school.html

MEDICAL SCHOOL, RESIDENCY, EXAMS

American Medical Schools requires applicants to show that they have done well in upper-level science courses, and on the MCAT exam, to ensure the matriculant can handle rigorous Medical School coursework. The application is standard and national, for all applicants. A few schools will require a secondary application. A personal interview will follow successful application. The interview is to determine if the applicant has the appropriate character, integrity and stamina, to thrive in a field of medicine.

Some schools try to identify those planning practice in poorly served specialties. Each Medical School takes a certain percentage of out-of-state applicants. This is particularly challenging in states where in-state matriculation is more competitive, such as New York and California. New York and California applicants can be therefore found throughout medical schools in the country.

Once accepted, the first two Medical School years are primarily classroom and laboratory education. This includes the dissection of a cadaver, in "gross laboratory" or "gross lab." Any school can vary, but most use the first year to deliver the advanced sciences, including histology, microbiology, anatomy and pharmacology. The second lecture year engages further into pathology, physiology and diseases. The 3rd and 4th years are clinical, mostly in the hospital, but also clinics and medical offices. The 4th year allows for some electives away from campus, and deeper exposures into the medical specialty or specialties being considered as a career.

Residency "Match" occurs the third Friday of March during the 4th medical school year. This is when the medical student discovers where they have matched for their on-the-job residency training. This Match occurs after the medical student has undergone another set of applications and interviews, this time at the prospective residency programs. The medical student will rank each of their residency selections, by preference as 1, 2, 3 and so on. Likewise, the residency program will rank their candidates by preference in an identical numerical order.

Unfortunately, there are a few medical students who do not match and have to scramble in securing a spot in a program that likewise did not match all their candidates. There is an attempt to create a balanced workforce. This is particularly true as doctor shortages are anticipated. There are certain residencies that are more competitive to secure. This can vary from year to year. Dermatology and Ophthalmology are a couple of these more perennially competitive residencies. This is likely because of the quieter office practice, better work-life balance and of course, compensation. Pediatric, Family Practice and Psychiatry have lower salaries compared to Surgeons and Specialists.

Those that were not selected into their residency specialty of choice can do a one-year internship and try again during the next Match. Some residents leave a residency voluntarily before completion or are "cut" (in other words, fired) from the residency. They may leave medicine altogether or go into another, oftentimes less stressful, residency. Residencies previously were more demanding. Many required overnight "call" or "on-call" every third or even every other night. Work hours were long and sleep was lacking. After all, "resident" historically meant living in the hospital. Even in the last few decades, it was not unusual for a resident to work 100 hours/week and 36 hours non-stop without sleep.

This grueling schedule was maintained until a certain event caught national attention. This event led to reform, first in New York, and then swept through the country into a national reform. In March 1984, 18-year-old Libby Zion died at New York Hospital from a medication error, while being cared for by residents on a 36-hour shift. An investigation led to passage of New York state regulations in 1987, capped resident work hour limits in New York hospitals, at 80 hours per week and no more than 24 consecutive hours. The rest of the country slowly caught on, even though there was plenty of resistance from some of the traditionally more demanding specialties, primarily surgery.

Further research began to show the correlation between fatigue and clinical performance. In 2003, the Accreditation Council for Graduate Medical Education (ACGME) adopted the New York model, and limited resident work hours to no more than 80 hours per week or 24 consecutive hours on duty. In addition, they required the resident not be "on-call" more than every third night, and have one day off each week. This regulation also eliminated extended-duration shifts for first-year residents. It should be recognized that we are not necessarily an international model for considerations of our medical trainees. Europe limits residents up to 48 duty hours per week.

Residents can complete training, get board certified, then acquire state licensure and begin a practice or employment. Some will go into further training in a higher-level residency or fellowship. For example, in order to train in Cardio-Thoracic Surgery, a medical student needs to complete a typical 5-year residency in General Surgery and then a typical 2-year residency in Cardio-Thoracic Surgery. There is a wide variety of further training in "fellowships" which can be a 1-year informal period to gain more experience or to become credentialed for a specialty board. Using our example, a resident who has completed 5 years of General Surgery residency can do an ICU fellowship and be "double-boarded" in both Surgery and Critical Care.

Residents are paid a salary and get benefits, just like most other U.S. employees. The current average annual salary for a resident is about $60,000. Many American college students incur loans to pay tuition and other living costs, during that education. Some can rack up very high debt. There is usually a 60-day grace period, before loan payments begin, after a higher education graduation. Medical students entering residencies can request loan forbearance.

Subsidized loans do not accrue interest with a forbearance during this time. Unsubsidized loans do accrue interest during forbearance. The resident can request a deferment at 12-month intervals, for military or fellowship placements.

Entering a residency is not the end of academic testing. It is actually the beginning of the tests that really matter. Passing these tests confer credentials of competencies on a doctor to, freely and legally, practice medicine and surgery.

The standard national medical licensing exam is actually three exams. It is called the United States Medical Licensing Examination (USMLE). The first exam, called Step 1, is given during the second year of Medical School. Step 1 covers the sciences fundamental to the practice of medicine. The Step 2 exam, which measures clinical knowledge and skills, is usually completed during the third or fourth year of Medical School. The final exam for initial licensure, Step 3, occurs during the first or second year of residency training, after completing medical school and receiving a medical degree.

Doctors of Osteopathy (DO) tend to choose primary care specialties, while allopathic medical doctors (MD) often enter specialty and urban practices. Caribbean medical school is another path. Certain characteristics of these medical schools and training will influence practice choices. But, for any ardent medical student, the sky is the limit.

References and Links
https://www.aamc.org/

https://www.usmle.org/

MD, DO, CARIBBEAN

Americans can go to Medical School either in the U.S., the Caribbean or overseas. Those that stay in the U.S., can attend one of two types of Medical Schools to become either an MD (Medical Doctor) or DO (Doctor of Osteopathy). More than 2/3 of all physicians in the U.S. are MDs. Seven percent are DOs. The remaining 25% get their Medical School training outside the U.S. Many of these trained outside enter Caribbean Medical Schools. It is more competitive to get an MD degree compared to a DO.

Becoming an MD requires higher average MCAT scores and GPAs (average 3.7), when compared to those becoming Dos (about 3.5). Caribbean Medical students have average GPAs and MCAT scores even lower than DOs. Those entered into Caribbean schools have GPAs averaging 3.2-3.4. This competitive hierarchy is also seen in residency-match results. MDs will match into U.S. residency programs at just over 90%, DOs at around 80% and Caribbean students at about a 50% match.

MD prospective applicants apply through the Association of American Medical Colleges (AAMC) into a Medical School that is accredited with the Liaison Committee on Medical Education (LCME). Prospective DOs apply through the American Association of Colleges of Osteopathic Medicine (AACOM) which also accredits their programs. Application to Caribbean schools is made directly to each school. All programs require the MCAT be taken prior to matriculation. All MD, DO and Caribbean Medical Schools require 4 years of Medical School education. All schools allow graduates to train and practice in any specialty anywhere in the U.S. DO Medical Schools require additional training in osteopathic manipulative medicine.

Caribbean Medical Schools are bastions for those American students who often don't get past the MCAT or GPA cut-offs for American-based Medical Schools, but are still good prospects to become physicians. Only 41% of applicants through the AAMC process get into an American-based MD school. Caribbean schools are often eligible for US Department of Education Title IV funding. This means that these students can receive federal financial aid. Caribbean schools typically offer merit scholarships. St. George's University is on the island of Grenada, in the West Indies. Ross University is in the Barbados. American University of the Caribbean, in French/Dutch Saint Maarten, is also regarded highly in this group. These three Caribbean medical schools, plus Saba Medical School on the island of Saba near St. Maarten, make up the so-called "Big Four." There are about 55-60 other Caribbean Medical Schools, including those less travelled in Cuba, Haiti and Jamaica. Most of these are taught in English. Many others are taught in Spanish.

American MD Schools have about a 4% attrition rate. This means 96% complete American Medical School training and go into residencies. In contrast, Ross University has a 20% drop out rate. One third of Caribbean medical students extend training beyond 4 years. U.S. MD schools have tuition that ranges from

$20,000 per semester for public in-state to nearly $70,000 per semester for public out-of-state or private medical schools. DO school tuition is very similar to MD schools. Caribbean Medical Schools average around $10,000 to $20,000 each semester. Added scholastic costs and fees will raise this cost of attending significantly further.

There are some unique aspects of Caribbean Schools. One can apply and enter into a Caribbean Medical School anytime through the year, through a rolling admission. In contrast, MD and DO schools start as 4-year cohorts each fall. The best Caribbean schools are accredited by the World Federation for Medical Education. Caribbean Medical School students must rotate at U.S. hospitals. This is done through agreements these schools have with American hospitals, as well as electives completed in other varied American hospitals.

Caribbean medical students must work hard to achieve a high GPA, score high on the USMLE and secure prestigious rotations at U.S. hospitals, in order to have the best odds of getting a better residency position. Educational Commission for Foreign Medical Graduates (ECFMG) certification is required of all foreign medical school graduates, before entering Accreditation Council for Graduate Medical Education (ACGME) residency or fellowship programs in the United States. This is an uphill battle. Two thirds of U.S. residency programs have indicated that they seldom or never interview to match international medical graduates, even though they are U.S. citizens. Some states have stricter guidelines and do not allow non-U.S. trained medical students and residents, to practice in that state. An American Medical School makes the transition into an American medical career much easier. But this can be well acquired even with Caribbean or other foreign medical education and training.

References and Links
https://www.ama-assn.org/residents-students/preparing-medical-school/do-vs-md-how-much-does-medical-school-degree-type
https://www.usnews.com/education/best-graduate-schools/top-medical-schools/articles/what-to-know-about-caribbean-medical-schools
https://www.acgme.org/
https://www.ecfmg.org/

LICENSING

Beginning on their first day, residents are licensed to practice medicine through a limited training certificate. This is a form of license issued to graduate physicians in accredited residency programs that permits them to practice under the supervision of fully licensed physicians. This extends until completion of the residency and application toward full state licensure. Some residents secure full licensure in order to moonlight during residency. Other training programs may require a resident physician to be fully licensed, at a certain point in that training. Full licensure varies with each state, but all require accredited education and training. One must pass a three-step test called the United States Medical Licensing Examination (USMLE), also known as the board exam, before applying for any state medical license.

The USMLE is a three-step examination sponsored by the Federation of State Medical Boards (FSMB) and the National Board of Medical Examiners (NBME). Physicians with an MD degree must pass this examination, in other words each and all of the three Step exams, before being permitted to practice Medicine in the United States. Students of Osteopathic Medicine, DOs, can take either the USMLE or a similar test called the Comprehensive Osteopathic Medical Licensing Examination (COMLEX). US citizens educated at Caribbean Medical Schools also need to take the USMLE. That is in addition to Educational Commission for Foreign Medical Graduates (ECFMG) certification.

Step 1 of the USMLE, currently scored on a numerical scale, will soon convert to pass/fail, like Step 2. Step 3 is still scored with a passing score threshold. USMLE Step 1, which is usually taken in the 2nd year of medical school, assesses whether medical school students or graduates understand and can apply the basic sciences to the practice of medicine.

USMLE Step 2, which is divided into Clinical Knowledge and Clinical Skills exams, applies the tenets of clinical sciences and patient-centered skills that provide for the safe and capable practice of medicine, in a supervised setting. This exam is typically taken during the 4th year of medical school. The final of the three USMLE exams, Step 3 ensures that the Medical student or graduate can apply medical knowledge and experience in the unsupervised practice of medicine. This last exam is usually taken after the first post-graduate year in residency. The USMLE will soon implement a reduction from 6 to 4 exam re-takes allowed for failed or incomplete Step or Step component attempts.

While every physician must be licensed to practice Medicine, Board Certification is a voluntary process. A Board Certificate is actually more than a feather in the cap. It has become a requirement to joining the staff of many U.S. hospitals, and a necessary requirement for many administrative medicine employments. Board Certifications are administered through the American Board of Medical Specialties. They all involve a competency examination. Fourteen medical specialty boards require an oral exam, in addition to the written, for initial certification. Like the USMLE,

Board Certification describes an individual physician with adequate and higher expertise and competence in that specialty. It has become, more or less, a standard. Board Certification requires updating on a 5-10-year basis. The boarded physician, for these Board Recertifications, must demonstrate specialty competency through similar examination, practice evaluation, continued education and good standing.

Each medical professional is licensed by each state of practice. This medical professional must apply separately in order to practice in another state or states. Many administrative physicians, and some clinical physicians, hold multiple state licenses in order to engage in utilization review and P2P interactions, and make medical necessity determinations, or engage in cross-state-border clinical practices. There is some uniformity and collection of data for state's licensure. The Interstate Medical Licensure Compact (IMLC) is a consortium of 29 participating states that agree to accept each other's vetting processes for medical licenses. Each of these states issues their own license. This is particularly important with the increases use of Telemedicine across states.

References and Links
https://www.ama-assn.org/residents-students/transition-practice/licensing-and-board-certification-what-residents-need-know
https://www.usmle.org/
https://www.nbome.org/
https://www.ecfmg.org/
https://www.abms.org/
https://www.imlcc.org/

NURSING

There are a few ways to become a nurse in the U.S. A typical three-semester training program can lead to certification as a Licensed Practical Nurse (LPN). There are some LPN programs that stretch longer into a degree. The LPN education is quicker than becoming a Registered Nurse (RN). Yet, an LPN will be restricted in professional activities. Salaries will be about half of that made by the typical RN. LPNs are licensed, just like RNs. The state boards licensing LPNs are usually the same state boards that license RNs. There are over 3,000,000 RNs and about 800,000 LPNs practicing now in the U.S. That is 4 RNs for every 1 LPN. There is greater demand for RNs over LPNs, because there is a greater demand for higher-level nurse positions and services. Both RNs and LPNs need to pass an examination in order to be licensed. The LPN needs to pass the National Council Licensure Examination, NCLEX-PN, while the RN needs to pass the NCLEX-RN.

The next level of nursing, above the LPN, is the Associate Degree Nurse (ADN) or Associate Degree RN. This is typically a 2-year program. This Nurse prospect will need to pass the NCLEX-RN for licensure. The Associate Degree RN will have the same full scope of practice as an RN. The incentive to go further to achieve a Bachelor Degree is because, although the Associate Degree nurse salary begins on the same scale as the RN, there is a quicker ceiling to advancement and pay for the ADN. Moving up the ladder into positions like management, leadership, or clinical nurse specialist are reserved for the RNs with baccalaureate degrees.

The baccalaureate degree RN is the highest standard educational level of the RN. Some RNs gain additional degrees such as Masters in Nursing or Master of Business Administration (MBA) or other related field advanced degrees. They then develop into nursing educators, such as college professors, or enter into hospital or other healthcare administration. These nurses even earn CEO positions of some hospitals and corporations.

There are a couple other variations on these pathways toward a nursing practice. There are some with a bachelor's degree in another field who did not initially seek to become a nurse. The accelerated bachelor's program requires the nurse prospect to fill in the prerequisite courses. These pre-requisites are typically algebra, geometry, chemistry and biology. Once those are satisfied, the student can then complete the remaining nursing courses at a faster pace.

As for all types of RN prospects, a strong GPA helps to secure a position in class. Again, as for all RNs, the NCLEX-RN is required before licensure. Many hospitals and nursing programs will allow the nursing student to engage in the Nurse Apprenticeship program. Although it doesn't shorten the education, it does allow the nursing student to work, and earn money and experience, while going through the RN education. Nursing is one of the best paying jobs in

America. It is in high demand while, at the same time, being demanding work.

References and Links
https://www.ncsbn.org/index.htm
https://nurse.org/education/types-of-nurses/

FOREIGN DOCTORS & NURSES

Doctors are increasingly being recruited, and also emigrate, from countries outside into the U.S. healthcare workforce. Doctors and nurses are coming from home countries of far lesser economies and much less economic support for their professional careers. About 1/3 of doctors practicing in the U.S. are foreign born and foreign trained. About 1 in 5 U.S. nurses are foreign born and foreign trained.

The majority of other foreign doctors come from the Philippines, China and India. Most go into under-served rural areas and primary care specialties, including psychiatry. That is because 70% of graduates of U.S. medical schools choose a specialty of practice and remain in hospital tertiary-care centers. Yet, there are a significant proportion of foreign doctors who are in higher-salaried specialties, such as cardiology, oncology and neurosurgery and some transition into hospital leadership and healthcare administrative positions. This move into administration makes way for even more foreign doctors to enter the US. The need for an increasing doctor workforce is following the aging of the Boomers. This will increase the need for foreign doctors, and all doctors, in the US.

By 2002, more than half of all physicians practicing in the U.S. had been educated and trained elsewhere. Many of these are Americans returning back after training in Caribbean Medical Schools and programs. Foreign-educated doctors must pass both the USMLE and ECFMG and then seek a J1 Visa. Those foreign nationals who have completed a U.S. residency must return to their home country for a two-year period of practice. That is, unless there is a hardship. They can then return back to a U.S. medical practice after this two-year-away interval.

An H-1B Visa allows a foreign doctor to enter the U.S. for employment for up to 6 years. This physician immigrant, who also must pass both USMLE and ECFMG exams, will have applied for and be granted an unrestricted U.S. state medical license to practice. A third option allowing foreign doctors to practice in the U.S. is with an immigrant visa, also called a green card or permanent resident status. It permits this foreign citizen to permanently remain in the U.S. practicing medicine. This green card holder has the right to become a naturalized U.S. citizen after living in this country for 5 years, or for 3 years if married to a U.S. citizen.

Every doctor, whether domestic or foreign, needs a U.S. state medical license to practice in that state. All states require a graduate of a foreign medical school to complete at least 1 year of accredited U.S. or Canadian graduate medical education before licensure. There are a dozen states that require 2 years, and twice that amount that require 3 years of accredited graduate medical education. Most hospitals will accept the ECFMG verified credentials of foreign education. But some hospitals require a direct transcript from that foreign medical school.

Completing a U.S. residency is the major hurdle for foreign doctors seeking to practice in the U.S. Only half are able to secure a residency. It is not unusual to have applied to residencies every year for several years until either finding success or simply giving up. Many U.S. residency programs require a preceding year of clinical experience in the U.S., completed within the last five years of foreign medical school graduation. Of course, these foreign candidates will need to score high on the USMLE and ECFMG exams, in order to gain notice.

Over 15% of U.S. nurses are foreign born. Over 1/3 of these foreign nurses come from the Philippines. The majority of nurses in U.S. nursing homes, and psychiatric aides in the U.S., come from Mexico and the Caribbean. Canadian nurses are driving over the US-Canadian border to practice in U.S. hospitals. Manila has several educational centers that filter Filipino nurses through the testing and into U.S. nursing homes, hospitals and medical offices. There is great financial incentive to make this move.

The foreign nurse has the added step of proving English proficiency, along with testing and accreditation and home-country practice, before eventually seeking a visa to practice nursing in the U.S. This immigration into the U.S. is only available for RNs and Advanced Practice Nurses (APN). LPNs, licensed vocational nurses, and patient care assistants (PCA) are not allowed to transfer their licenses to the U.S.

The foreign nurse must initially graduate from an accredited RN program and then be licensed in that country. The foreign RN then needs to practice for at least two years in their country. The foreign RN must prove English proficiency either by attending an English nursing school, being from an English-speaking country or passing either the Test of English as a Foreign Language (TOEFL), the Test of English for International Communication (TOEIC) or the International English Language Testing System (IELTS).

The foreign nurse has to pass the NCLEX, just like an American nurse. This exam is administered in Australia, Canada, England, Germany, Hong Kong, India, Japan, Mexico, the Philippines, Puerto Rico, and Taiwan. Before entry into the U.S., the foreign RN needs to undergo credentialing by the US-based Commission on Graduates of Foreign Nursing Schools (CGFNS). This includes visa credentialing. The foreign RN, upon satisfying the visa credentialing, will receive a certificate to the consular office in their country in order to apply for a visa to work in the U.S. These RNs can enter by a work-sponsored employment or "work" visa. Mexican and Canadian nurses can cross the border and practice through a TN Visa. Like foreign doctors, these foreign RNs can also practice on an H1 Visa or become permanent residents.

The financial incentives of immigrating into a U.S. healthcare profession far outweigh the hardships. As the U.S. population ages, there will be increased demand. That demand will continue to be satisfied by the flow of both domestic and foreign trained workers into healthcare professions.

References and Links

https://www.ama-assn.org/education/international-medical-education/practicing-medicine-us-international-medical-graduate

https://www.ncsbn.org/index.htm

https://www.cgfns.org/steps-to-working-as-nurse-in-united-states/

DOCTOR PRIVILEGES

Before practicing in a hospital, a doctor must become credentialed and granted privileges. Credentialing is the verification of education and training, board certification if required, and state licensure. Privileges are the scope of practice in that hospital. A doctor must have training and experience in a procedure or service in order to earn those requested privileges. For example, a Gastroenterologist (GI) will request privileges to admit and care for GI patients and also do endoscopies. Full or active hospital privileges are the entire scope granted for that specialty, along with all hospital activities. Courtesy privileges allow the doctor to occasionally admit patients and act as a consultant. These courtesy privileges do not allow one to participate in medical staff activities. Usually, every 2 years or so, a member of the hospital staff will undergo conduct appraisals for continued or revised hospital privileges.

Medical staff bylaws are created by medical staff and approved by the hospital governing board, describing the rights, responsibilities, and accountabilities of their medical staff. These rules include those that direct the credentialing, medical staff requirements and activities and privileges processes. They also describe the conduct and responsibilities of practicing in that hospital.

Denied privileges happen infrequently. It can happen when there is a deficiency in the credentials or there is identified misconduct or inadequate proficiency information. One example of denied privileges, is a candidate for family medicine privileges who may also request privileges to deliver babies. The hospital may require obstetrics/gynecology residency training to deliver babies. The privileges to deliver babies would be denied to that family practice physician. While other appropriate training and experience related privileges may would be granted to this family practitioner.

Denied privileges gives the applicant the right to a fair hearing. These can be expensive for the hospital. So, the denial needs to be on firm grounds. The physician should be granted privileges that are appropriate for their specialty, training and experience. They should not be denied privileges based on personal, political or workforce issues.

References and Links

http://www.hpso.com/risk-education/individuals/articles/Staff-Credentialing-Checklist

https://www.abpsus.org/hospital-privileges/

https://www.ama-assn.org/delivering-care/ethics/staff-privileges

https://www.jointcommission.org/standards/standard-faqs/hospital-and-hospital-clinics/medical-staff-ms/000002124/

REGULATORY & LEGAL

HOSPITAL
CREDENTIALING

Hospitals can be accredited by one of several difference organizations. Being accredited and certified, means the facility is engaging in best practices and minima quality standards. Accreditation can be from URAC (Utilization Review Accreditation Commission), NCQA (National Committee for Quality Assurance), TJC (The Joint Commission), CARF (Commission on Accreditation of Rehabilitation Facilities) or COA (Council on Accreditation). Most hospitals and clinics get accreditation from TJC. Accreditation by TJC is considered the gold standard. The majority of hospitals most highly ranked by US News Best Hospitals, Watson/Truven Health Analytics, Healthgrades America's Best Hospitals, Baldridge National Quality Award recipients and Magnet status hospitals are accredited by TJC. TJC accreditation is sought for even international facilities, as well as physician offices, nursing homes, office-based surgery centers, behavioral health treatment facilities and providers of home care services.

Hospitals earn accreditation for several doing business in healthcare, quality and standardization reasons. They also need accreditation to receive payment from federally funded Medicare and Medicaid programs. TJC accredits more than 4,000 US facilities, which is 78% of all hospitals throughout the country. Other agencies accredit another 11% of US hospitals. The remaining 11% of US hospitals do not undergo any accreditation. Some of these may be specialty hospitals or clinics. Other hospitals are instead choosing ISO (International Organization for Standardization) instead of traditional accreditation. ISO registration is an international standards program that is common in manufacturing. ISO certification allows these hospitals to participate in both the Medicare/Medicaid programs and in many insurance programs. Although hospital accreditation is voluntary, it is in the hospital's best interest to maintain high standards and demonstrate and display to the public, this though industry accreditation.

References and Links
https://www.jointcommission.org/
https://www.urac.org/
https://www.ncqa.org/
https://www.iso.org/caring-about-health-and-safety.html

CERTIFICATE OF NEED (CON)

Certificate of Need (CON) regulations are intended to control costs and healthcare inflation by limiting healthcare facility capacity within a state or community. The first CON regulation was enacted into New York state law in 1964, through the Metcalf–McCloskey Act. The Act intends to promote cost containment, prevent duplicitous healthcare facilities and services, and direct the establishment of health facilities and services to serve the need and promote improved quality services. Another 18 states followed New York's lead up to the time of the federally enacted Section 1122 of the Social Security Act in 1972. Now 37 states have CON laws. Twenty two of these 37 states did reduce or rescind their CON laws when greater resources were needed during the COVID-19 pandemic.

Hospital beds are fixed costs. Hospitals raise the fixed costs on occupied beds in order to cover their empty non-revenue beds. This is particularly true with larger hospitals and hospital systems. This increased revenue pays for more facilities, further increasing healthcare costs. CON programs require a healthcare facility to demonstrate to a health planning agency, that there is a community need for that facility. That health planning agency may approve, deny or set certain limitations on the healthcare project. The notion is that more affordable healthcare services will be accessed by the rightsizing of healthcare. CON programs are an effective way to control healthcare costs and in this way increase access to more patients.

Critics of the CON programs see them as unnecessary barriers to entry into the market for smaller or individual systems, by protecting established and larger health facilities already in that market. It has been suggested by some that CON may, paradoxically, decrease competition and lead to increases in healthcare prices. CON laws vary from state to state, creating complexities in the planning for national healthcare facilities.

Politics can influence a state CON decision. The U.S. economy can wax and wane. CONs are less nimble in predicting and following economic trends to maintain facility numbers which must serve that community for years and decades to come. Healthcare inflation was high, at 13% during the late 1960s to the early 1980s. Those were the prime years for supporting the CON. Healthcare inflation then dropped to about 1.5% during the end of 2017 and through 2019. Now we are currently at 5%. This changing economic climate weakens the central argument for CON. It needs to be determined whether CONs still have justification or are a good-intentioned vestige of a bygone era.

References and Links
https://www.ncsl.org/research/health/con-certificate-of-need-state-laws.aspx
https://www.ncbi.nlm.nih.gov/pmc/articles/PMC7427974/

INSURANCE COMMISSIONS

An insurance commissioner, as an executive public official, regulates the insurance industry in that U.S. state or territory. Most insurance commissioners are appointed, while others are elected. All insurance commissioners are members of the National Association of Insurance Commissioners (NAIC). Insurance laws and regulations can vary in each state. The NAIC has model laws and statutes that each state can use for their own insurance regulations.

The job of the insurance commissioner is a balance between the protection of the public while fostering a broad and fair insurance industry. The insurance commissioner ensures the availability of fair-priced insurances and prevents unfair practices. They have the power to approve insurance rates, monitor and regulate insurance claims, license insurance companies, agencies, agents and brokers and examine the finances of each insurer.

Any complaint or concern by a state's healthcare beneficiary of that agency or agent, or its delegates, would be directed to the state insurance commissioner. This turns out to be a big stick for many insurers or their vendors, since that insurance commissioner has the power to ultimately remove that insurer from the state's marketplace.

References and Links

https://content.naic.org/

NATIONAL PRACTITIONERS DATA BANK

A medical or nursing state license is required of every U.S. practitioner. A practitioner must maintain good standing in order to keep and renew a state professional license. Malpractice claims and outcomes, and regulatory or insurance complaints from the public, are situations that may impact good standing.

The National Practitioner Data Bank (NPDB) was established by Congress in 1968 to promote quality healthcare and combat fraud and abuse within healthcare delivery. The NPDB does this by collecting and distributing reports of medical malpractice payments and adverse actions attributed to healthcare practitioners, providers, suppliers and healthcare organizations. The data points that the NPDB collects are medical malpractice pay-outs, adverse clinical privilege events, adverse professional society membership events, adverse licensure and certification actions, negative actions by peer review and civil judgments and criminal convictions in federal or state courts.

A primary purpose of the NPDB is to prevent practitioners from moving state-to-state without revealing any and all previous adverse events. Eligible entities, such as hospitals, insurance commissioners, professional associations and others, are required to submit their information to the NPDB. These same entities, as well as the practitioners who are being reported, are able to query this data set. Yet, these reports are considered confidential and not fully available to the public. The public only has access to broad statistical data, which does not identify individuals.

References and Links
https://www.npdb.hrsa.gov/

FEDERAL FRAUD LAWS

The Office of Inspector General of the U.S. Department of Health and Human Services enforces five fraud and abuse laws which apply to physicians and health services, under federal jurisdiction. These are the False Claims Act (FCA), the Anti-Kickback Statute (AKS), the Physician Self-Referral Law (Stark law), the Exclusion Authorities, and the Civil Monetary Penalties Law (CMPL).

The civil False Claims Act protects against overcharging or charging for absent or incomplete Medicare or Medicaid goods or services. These false charges for goods or services are known, or should have been known, to be false or fraudulent. No specific provider intent to defraud is required. "Knowing" means actually knowing or even deliberate ignorance or reckless disregard of the truth or falsity of the information. Fines for this fraud can be up to three times the loss plus $11,000 per claim filed. There are also criminal penalties of imprisonment and criminal fines, for submitting false claims. The civil FCA contains a whistleblower provision, allowing a percentage of any recovery.

A healthcare provider cannot induce or reward referral to itself for any Medicare or Medicaid program, under the Anti-Kickback Statute. This is a criminal law that prohibits the knowing and willful payment, by both the giver and recipient. Illegal remuneration for referral can be cash, discounts of rent, excessive salary for phony positions, or gifts including expensive travel. Neither harm, financial loss nor incomplete service, even if that service is medically necessary, needs to be show for a violation of this statute to occur. Penalties include fines up to $50,000 per kickback plus three times the amount of the remuneration, jail terms, and exclusion from participation in the federal healthcare programs.

There are some very narrow safe-harbor relationship protections under this law, including personal services and rental agreements, investments in ambulatory surgical centers, and payments to bona fide employees, that would otherwise be considered illegal renumeration. Waiving a copay for a Medicare or Medicaid recipient can be done on an individual and compassionate basis. Otherwise, a uniformly waived copay, or one that was advertised to do so, would be a violation of the AKS.

It is illegal for physicians, under the Physician Self-Referral Law, also called the Stark law, to refer patients to designated services payable to Medicare and Medicaid, with which either that physician or an immediate family member has a financial relationship. These specific and designated prohibited self-referral services are through their laboratories, therapies, imaging, nutrition, inpatient, home and outpatient services The troublesome financial relationships include ownership, investment and compensation arrangements. That is, unless that enriching arrangement is considered a "safe harbor" under this statute.

The most prominent example of a Stark law violation that in fact lead to these laws, were physician-owned blood drawing labs that were set up within their offices. There was a conspicuous over ten times increase in laboratory testing immediately after physicians began to put in these labs. The Stark law is a strict liability statute which does not require proof of specific intent to violate this law. The provider doesn't need to realize that it is a violation, for a violation to occur. The Stark law prohibits the submission, or causing the submission, of claims in violation of the law's restrictions on referrals. Penalties are fines and exclusions from participation in the federal healthcare programs.

Physicians and providers are excluded, through the federal Exclusion Statute, from all federal healthcare programs if convicted of these and other related criminal offenses. These exclusionary actions are due to Medicare or Medicaid fraud or abuse through the named statutes and acts, as well as other offenses against those programs, patient abuse or neglect, felony convictions for other health-care-related fraud, theft or other financial misconduct, and unlawful manufacture, distribution, prescription, or dispensing of controlled substances. The federal government is intent on paying fairly and only paying for appropriate goods and services rendered. Despite these penalties and monitoring, abuse against these programs remains high.

References and Links

https://oig.hhs.gov/compliance/physician-education/

https://oig.hhs.gov/fraud/index.asp

https://www.cms.gov/Outreach-and-Education/Medicare-Learning-Network-MLN/MLNProducts/Downloads/Fraud-Abuse-MLN4649244.pdf

MEDICAL MALPRACTICE & DEFENSIVE MEDICINE

Medical malpractice occurs when a facility or healthcare professional causes an injury to a patient due to a negligent act or omission. The plaintiff launching this lawsuit is often the patient or family (estate). The defendant targets, as stated, are the providers, doctors and/or healthcare facilities. Negligence can be due to errors in diagnosis, treatment, or the subsequent health management.

A medical malpractice claim can be brought if the doctor violates the standard of care, causing an injury that results in significant damages. The standard that the provider should follow is acceptable medical treatment by reasonably prudent healthcare professionals, under like or similar circumstances. The injury must occur from a violation of that standard of care. The injury must cause disability, a loss of income, unusual pain, suffering and hardship, or incur significant past and future medical bills. There is no claim if the injury would have occurred without the negligence. Every unfavorable outcome or complication are not due to negligence.

The injury must be significant enough to translate into a substantial money equivalent. Medical malpractice lawsuits are expensive to litigate, since they require recruiting numerous medical experts and hours of deposition testimony. The cost of the case could end up being greater than a small award. So, attorneys are adept at identifying potentials winners in settlements or the rare case that will go to trial. These attorneys have been accused of bringing too many frivolous lawsuits to determine which of them will stick. The majority of states' jurisdictions have regulations against obvious frivolous lawsuits.

Most attorneys will work with a contingency agreement. This means the plaintiff pays nothing unless there is an award. That award to the injured medical malpractice party is reduced by the contingency amount that is shared with the attorney(s). This contingency is usually a 40% cut of the award for those attorneys. Most often the costs of this litigation, which include expert medical witness fees, and discovery of records and court filing fees, will be reimbursed to the attorneys initially from the award total. This arrangement reduces the total award to the injured. For example, a 60/40 contingency agreement with a $100,000 settlement and $20,000 in litigation costs would leave the injured with ($100,000 - $20,000 = $80,000 x .6) $48,000. Malpractice awards are not considered income and are not federally taxed.

Currently, there are over 10,000 medical malpractice claims paid each year, for close to $4 billion. New York, New Jersey, Pennsylvania and Florida have the highest amount of paid medical malpractice claims and the highest premiums for malpractice insurance. The Institute of Medicine (IOM) estimates that between 44,000 and 98,000 patients die in hospitals annually from preventable medical errors. Many believe this is gross undercounting and see it as 4-5 times higher. The IOM positions these hospital error deaths as the 6th leading cause of overall deaths in the US. The medical malpractice proponents believe it is actually higher, as the 3rd cause of death in Americans. Yet, even with these rates, less than 5% of victims of medical malpractice bring a suit. This is either because they are not aware, or not confident that the untoward event was negligence, or because they don't seek retribution on their caregivers.

Some of the more common specific medical malpractice claims would be failure to diagnose or misdiagnosis, wrong-side or wrong-site surgery, incorrect medication or dosage and failure to order proper testing. The typical medical malpractice lawsuit starts with filing of the case with the court and service of a summons and complaint to the defendant. Both parties then do discovery through which medical records are exchanged, and depositions are taken from the parties and witnesses. The case may be dismissed by the judge, settled out-of-court with a monetary settlement or go to court with a jury trial or to a specialized health court. More than 90% of all medical malpractice settles out of court, either because there is apparent medical error or because one or both parties wants to avoid the high cost of court proceedings. Some suggest that this promotes the bringing of frivolous lawsuits.

Through the practice of defensive medicine, doctors try to avoid a medical malpractice lawsuit. Defensive medicine is leaving no-stone-unturned in the evaluation of a patient's complaint, with overuse and over-utilization of medical tests and procedures. A medical malpractice claim leaves a doctor feeling defeated. They often go into depression, change their practice style or even change careers. Some even take their own lives. The medical malpractice litigation process takes an average of 2-3 years. During this time, the doctor is second guessing each patient. They are devoting their lives to caring for other people as patients, only to become a financial and legal target.

Defensive medicine is a perceived strategy to lessen becoming that medical malpractice target. It has been shown that up to 60% of all healthcare costs are attributable to the low-value-added high cost of defensive medicine. The excessive tests and procedures associated with defensive medicine may theoretically protect from medical malpractice claim, but at a high cost. Over-utilization can lead to unintentional iatrogenic injuries and the cascading costs of more and more evaluations. Defensive medicine, distinct from true medical necessity, adds extra costs into the healthcare system. These extra costs are ultimately paid by the patient through higher fees and premiums.

Tort reform has been the most common tactic to control the doctor's claims of runaway medical malpractice. These laws vary by jurisdiction, primarily imposed by state jurisdictions. Tort reform reduces either, or both, the ability of victims to litigate and the damages they can receive with successful litigation. The majority of states have imposed variable amounts of caps on medical malpractice claims. These caps vary across the states, and state laws may frequently change. Tort reform is not wider sweeping because attorneys argue that the injured should be made whole, and that actual medical malpractice should be punished. Attorneys, along with those holding political offices who are mostly attorneys themselves, are a strong and influential force against tort reform. Instead, improved safety has been addressed through provider or hospital directed time-outs, correct side and surgery confirmations and other team practices and fail-safes to ensure safe and diligent healthcare.

References and Links

https://www.ncbi.nlm.nih.gov/pmc/articles/PMC2628513/

https://www.ncsl.org/research/health/medical-malpractice-reform-health-cost-brief.aspx

https://www.policymed.com/2010/09/defensive-medicine-adds-45-billion-to-the-cost-of-healthcare.html

https://physicianlitigationstress.org/coping-with-litigation/

https://www.medscape.com/viewarticle/418841_1

Most of the public is aware that there is confidentiality, also called a privilege in the communications between a lawyer and client. This privilege also exists between a husband and wife, as well as a doctor and patient. Likewise, there are confidentiality protections for documents and communications generated during a review of a doctor's behavior and actions, within a peer review committee.

The Federal Patient Safety and Quality Improvement Act (PSQIA) privilege allows a provider to voluntarily provide information on adverse medical events that are protected from being used as evidence in a medical malpractice action. This evidentially privilege under federal law, is for this patient safety work product given to a certified Patient Safety Organization (PSO). This pre-empts any State peer review privilege laws, when there is federal-question jurisdiction.

The Peer Review Protection Act ("PRPA") of 1974 gives limited immunity and confidentiality to healthcare providers who, through post-care review and investigation, try to improve the quality of patient care. The PRPA provides limited immunity protection against disclosure to those involved in the peer review process, as well as documents and communications generated as part of that peer review process. The peer review group must have as its purpose and goals improving the quality of care rendered, reducing morbidity and mortality, establishing and enforcing policies of cost containment, reviewing qualifications for medical staff and reviewing the operations of their facilities. But these protections only extend to that information which is created because of this review. Documents and communications that would not be protected under this act include original source information, even if later submitted to the peer review committee, business records, patient safety incident reports and physician applications for staff privileges. Conversely, information protected would be "root cause analysis" or analysis of "sentinel events," the physician's NPDB file and any communication to the plaintiff indicating that the peer review concluded there was no failure to meet standard of care. Yet, protections under PRPA can be waived when the peer review documents are transferred to defense counsel or facility risk management, in order to prepare a defense for a deposition.

All 50 states and the District of Columbia, have passed statutes to protect peer review communications and documents and give immunity to those engaging in the peer review process. In addition, there are federal and state mandates to establish peer review committees in order to receive federal funding for Medicare and Medicaid. TJC now requires hospitals to establish peer review of medical staff.

There are some elements of these laws that are shared across many states. The Pennsylvania Peer Review Protection Act ("PRPA") is used as an example to illustrate these more common features. This law gives limited immunity and confidentiality to healthcare providers who, through post-care review and investigation, try to improve the quality of patient care. The PRPA provides limited immunity protection against disclosure to those involved in the peer review process, as well as documents and communications generated as part of that peer review process. The peer review group must have as its purpose and goals improving the quality of care rendered, reducing morbidity and mortality, establishing and enforcing policies of cost containment, reviewing qualifications for medical staff and reviewing the operations of their facilities. But these protections only extend to that information which is created because of this review. Documents and communications that would not be protected under this act include original source information, even if later submitted to the peer review committee, business records, patient safety incident reports and physician applications for staff privileges. Conversely, information protected would be root cause analysis or analysis of sentinel events, the physician's NPDB file and any communication to the plaintiff indicating that the peer review concluded there was no failure to meet standard of care. Yet, protections under PRPA can be waived when the peer review documents are transferred to defense counsel or facility risk management, in order to prepare a defense for a deposition.

Peer review is intended for providers to police their own. To improve when errors are identified. They are given confidentiality tools to do this, by both the federal and state regulations, to go forward reasonably, fairly and to protect the safety of American patients.

References and Links

https://www.hhs.gov/hipaa/for-professionals/patient-safety/statute-and-rule/index.html

https://www.legis.state.pa.us/WU01/LI/LI/US/PDF/1996/0/0142..PDF

PRE-EXISTING CONDITION

The pre-existing condition clause, often found in health plans as recent as before the passage of the ACA, would cancel coverage for certain known conditions during a waiting period. Insurers would not pay any claims for services rendered for that condition, until after the beneficiary had waited through a specific time period. The pre-existing condition exclusion was a way for insurers to seek a lower-risk lower-cost pool. Since high-risk individuals with pre-existing conditions would have barriers to signing up and accessing that health insurance.

Chronic illness in Americans is not at all unusual. Over 60% of Americans have one chronic health condition, with 40% having multiple chronic illnesses. The leading chronic conditions are heart disease, cancer, chronic lung disease, stroke, Alzheimer's Disease, diabetes and chronic kidney disease. Other pre-existing conditions can include epilepsy, lupus, inflammatory bowel disease, and even acne, depression, anxiety and pregnancy.

During the early period, one could get the pre-existing condition exclusion waived with demonstration of preceding credible health insurance coverage. The credible coverage could only be terminated up to 63 days before joining the current health plan. Prior to the ACA and through the 1990s, Massachusetts, followed by Maine, New Jersey, New

York and Vermont required health insurers to cover any patient, regardless of a pre-existing condition. The HIPAA enactment in 1997 set this maximum amount of wait at 12 months, or 18 months for late enrollees. All the while during this wait, the subscribers would still need to pay monthly premiums and could receive other services through the plan. Health plans could even refuse to cover a prospective subscriber with a pre-existing condition.

Under the ACA law beginning on January 1, 2014, health insurers could no longer refuse coverage or charge more for any pre-existing condition. The insurer also could not refuse to cover treatment for a pre-existing condition, even after the member signed up for that plan. Now, more than a dozen states have laws that would preserve key ACA pre-existing condition protections if the federal law is overturned. The vast majority of Americans, up to 85%, express their support for the pre-existing condition exclusion and never want to see it return in their lifetimes.

References and Links

https://www.hhs.gov/healthcare/about-the-aca/pre-existing-conditions/index.html

https://www.cms.gov/CCIIO/Resources/Forms-Reports-and-Other-Resources/preexisting

https://www.commonwealthfund.org/blog/2020/state-efforts-preexisting-conditions

ABOUT THE AUTHOR

A major near-death illness while uninsured during medical
school, impressed the author with the challenges and
wonders of American healthcare. He engaged initially in
clinical surgical practice, then administrative healthcare,
over the course of a 25-year career. His writings are
instructional, informative and revealing based on the
meta-present American healthcare system. For which he
has been a contributor and participant, through profession
and lifelong illness. He sees our healthcare as aggravating
and costly, but at the same time, uniquely hopeful,
transformative and treasured.